Lite Delight

300 Calories or Less!

PUBLICATIONS INTERNATIONAL, LTD.

Campbell's, V8, and Swanson are registered trademarks of the Campbell Soup Company.

Pictured on the front cover (*clockwise from top right*): Creamy Lemon Cheesecake (*page 79*), Apricot Muffins (*page 26*), Minestrone (*page 30*) and Herb-Marinated Chicken Breast (*page 38*) served with Bacon Pilaf (*page 66*).

Pictured on the back cover (*clockwise from top right*): Banana Bran Loaf (*page 31*), Springtime Vegetable Slaw (*page 70*) and Scandinavian Smörgåsbord (*page 11*).

ISBN 1-56173-086-6
Library of Congress Catalog Card Number: 90-63050

This edition published by:
Publications International, Ltd.
7373 N. Cicero Avenue
Lincolnwood, IL 60646

Printed and bound in Yugoslavia
9 8 7 6 5 4 3 2 1

Microwave cooking times in this book are approximate. Numerous variables, such as the microwave oven's rated output wattage and the starting temperature, shape, type, and amount and depth of food, can affect cooking time. Use the cooking times as guidelines and check doneness before adding more time. Lower wattage ovens may require longer cooking times.

Lite Delight

INTRODUCTION   4

Helping you make smart decisions about the foods you choose to prepare.

APPETIZERS & BEVERAGES   6

Light hors d'oeuvres perfect for any party, plus plenty of both hot and cold drinks to choose from.

SOUPS & BREADS   20

A collection of main-dish and starter soups, along with a wonderful selection of breads and muffins.

MAIN DISHES   34

Enjoy a variety of main dishes with these wonderful meat, fish, poultry and pasta entrées.

SALADS & SIDE DISHES   58

A wonderful array of hearty lunch-time salads, light side-dish salads, salad dressings and vegetable side-dishes.

DESSERTS   74

The perfect indulgence: low calorie, low fat desserts that taste great.

ACKNOWLEDGMENTS   92

INDEX   93

Introduction

Finally, You Can Have It All

Like most people, you've probably had enough of all those empty-calorie, high-fat fast foods. You want to make better choices about the foods you eat, but you don't want to spend a lot of time or trouble preparing meals that taste good and are good for you. Finally, it's all right here at your fingertips. For the first time here's a collection of recipes that are not only low in calories, fat and cholesterol, but are also easy to prepare *and* sure to taste good because they all use products and brands that you've come to trust.

Everyone's concerned with calories, fat, cholesterol and sodium. Studies declare that most Americans are overweight and that the American diet is loaded with too much fat and "empty calories" — calories from high-fat, high-sugar fast foods or snack foods that supply few necessary nutrients. Other studies have shown a clear link between a poor diet and heart disease. As a result, Americans are waking up to the fact that a poor diet can lead to poor health. Food producers and manufacturers are waking up to this trend as well. Supermarkets now regularly stock leaner cuts of beef and pork. The freezer cases feature frozen convenience foods that are low in calories, fat, cholesterol and sodium. And most people are aware of the extraordinary number of new products making all manner of health claims.

But many of these claims are misleading while others are still the subject of scientific debate. The average consumer is left confused. What constitutes low-calorie? Low-fat? What's good for you? What isn't? The American Heart Association has offered guidelines to help people adjust their diets to try to prevent heart and vascular diseases and we've followed those guidelines in choosing the recipes for this book.

Making Smart Choices

The recipes that follow can help you make smart, healthy decisions about the foods you prepare. Every recipe in this book is followed by a nutritional chart that tells you the number of calories, the grams (g) of fat, the milligrams (mg) of cholesterol and the milligrams of sodium for each serving of that recipe. To be considered for this book recipes had to contain 300 calories or less per serving, and contain no more than 10 grams of fat per serving.

Many of the recipes in this book are low-cholesterol and low-sodium as well. These recipes contain less than 50 mg of cholesterol and less than 300 mg of sodium. As you browse through the book you'll see that most of the recipes fall well below these numbers. In addition, many recipes are especially quick and easy to prepare, requiring 30 minutes or less in the kitchen. You can easily find these recipes by looking for the color bars below each recipe title:

Low Cholesterol

Low Sodium

Quick & Easy

The values of 300 calories, 10 g of fat, 50 mg cholesterol and 300 mg sodium per serving, were chosen after careful consideration of a number of factors. The Food and Nutrition Board of the National Academy of Sciences proposes the Recommended Dietary Allowances (RDAs) for all nutritive components including calories, carbohydrates, fat, protein, amino acids, vitamins and minerals. The RDAs were most recently revised in 1989. The RDA for calories is broken down according to age groups and sex. For men between the ages of 19 and 50, for example, the RDA for total calorie intake is 2,900 calories per day. For women between the ages of 19 and 50, it is 2,200 calories per day. Thus, the 300 calories or less per serving for the recipes in this book represents only about 10 percent of the RDA for most men and about 14 percent of the RDA for most women.

The American Heart Association has recommended that total fat intake should be less than 30 percent of calories. For most women that amounts to about 660 calories from fat (or about 73 grams of fat) per day; for most men about 870 calories or about 97 grams of fat per day. Thus the 10 grams of fat or less per serving for each recipe in this book is well within recommended guidelines. The American Heart Association also recommends that cholesterol intake be less than 300 mg a day and sodium intake not exceed 3,000 mg a day. The numbers we chose for recipes to be considered low-cholesterol (50 mg or less) or low-sodium (300 mg or less) are also well within these guidelines.

About the Nutritional Information

The analysis of each recipe includes all the ingredients that are listed in that recipe, except ingredients labelled as "optional" or "for garnish." If a range is given in the yield of a recipe ("Makes 6 to 8 servings," for example), the *higher* yield was used to calculate the per serving information. If a range is offered for an ingredient (¼ to ⅛ teaspoon, for example) the *first* amount given was used to calculate the nutrition information. If an ingredient is presented with an option ("2 tablespoons margarine or butter") the *first* item listed was used to calculate the nutrition information. Foods shown in photographs on the same serving plate and offered as "serve with" suggestions at the end of a recipe are *not* included in the recipe analysis unless it is stated in the per serving line.

The nutrition information that appears with each recipe was submitted by the participating companies and associations. **Every effort has been**

made to check the accuracy of these numbers. However, because numerous variables account for a wide range of values for certain foods, all nutritive analyses that appear in this book should be considered approximate. The numbers that appear in the nutrition charts are based on the nutritive values for foods in the U.S. Department of Agriculture Composition of Foods Handbook No. 8 (series), or from values submitted directly by the food·manufacturers themselves. (For more information, see the introductions to the Handbook No. 8 series.)

What This Book Does and Does Not Do

The recipes in this book were all selected to help you make smart choices about the foods you prepare. And with more than 180 recipes contributed by America's largest food companies, you'll find plenty to choose from. There are appetizers, beverages, soups and breads; meat, fish, poultry and pasta main dishes, salads, vegetable side dishes and desserts. From breakfast to dinner, from party fare to everyday meals, you can find wonderful, low-calorie, low-fat recipes to serve to family and friends.

This book offers you a wide variety of recipes that are, on a per serving basis, low in calories, fat and cholesterol. **The recipes in this book are NOT intended as a medically therapeutic program, nor as a substitute for medically approved diet plans for people on fat-, cholesterol- or sodium-restricted diets. You should consult your physician before beginning any diet plan.** The recipes offered here can be part of a healthy lifestyle that meets recognized dietary guidelines. A healthy lifestyle includes not only eating a balanced diet, but engaging in proper exercise as well.

By preparing foods that are low in calories, fat, cholesterol and sodium you can begin to enjoy a healthier lifestyle. And with all the wonderful dishes offered here you don't have to sacrifice either flavor or convenience. So start on the road to better living and great eating with this marvelous collection of low-calorie, low-fat recipes.

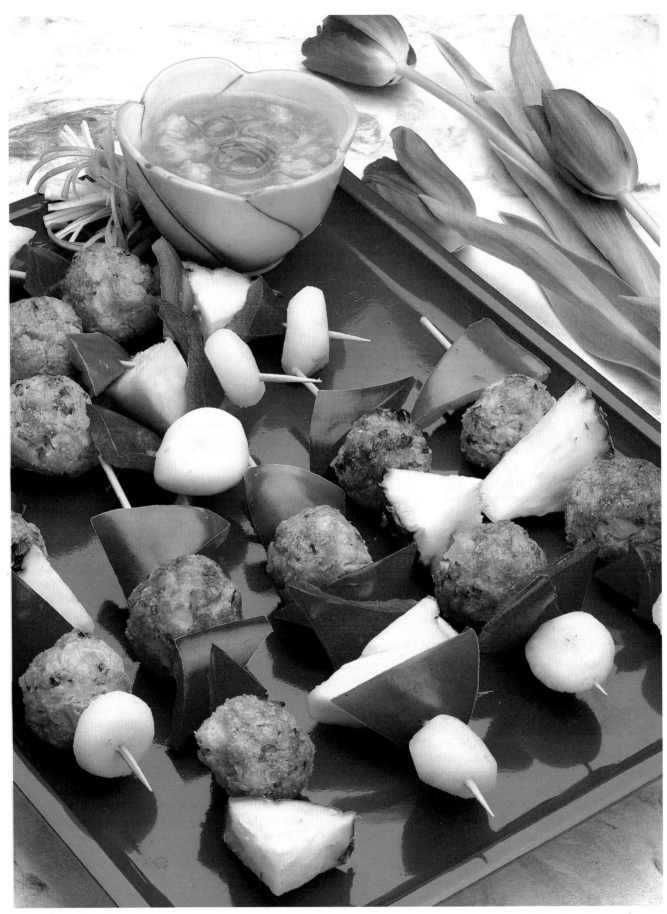

Appetizers & Beverages

Shanghai Party Pleasers

Low Sodium

Makes 2 dozen

1 can (20 oz.) crushed pineapple in juice,
   undrained
¼ cup firmly packed brown sugar
2 tablespoons cornstarch
   Dash of ginger
1 cup water
2 tablespoons margarine
1 pound finely chopped, cooked, skinned turkey
   or chicken
¾ cup QUAKER® Oat Bran hot cereal, uncooked
⅓ cup plain low fat yogurt
⅓ cup finely chopped water chestnuts, drained
⅓ cup sliced green onions
2 tablespoons lite soy sauce
1 egg white, slightly beaten
1 teaspoon ginger
½ teaspoon salt (optional)

Drain pineapple, reserving juice. In medium
saucepan, combine brown sugar, cornstarch and dash
of ginger; mix well. Add combined pineapple juice,
water, ¼ cup pineapple and margarine; mix well.
Bring to a boil over medium-high heat; reduce heat.
Simmer about 1 minute, stirring frequently or until
sauce is thickened and clear. Set aside.

Heat oven to 400°F. Lightly spray rack of 13×9-inch
baking pan with vegetable oil cooking spray or oil
lightly. Combine turkey, oat bran, yogurt, water
chestnuts, onions, soy sauce, egg white, 1 teaspoon
ginger, salt and remaining pineapple; mix well. Shape
into 1-inch balls. Place on prepared rack. Bake 20 to
25 minutes or until light golden brown. Serve with
pineapple sauce.

Nutrients per serving (⅛ of recipe):

Calories	240	Sodium	240 mg
Fat	6 g	Cholesterol	45 mg

Ginger Shrimp

Low Cholesterol

Makes about 2 dozen

1 cup (8 ounces) Lite WISH-BONE® Italian
   Dressing
½ cup sherry
4 medium shallots, peeled and halved°
3 medium green onions, cut into pieces
1 (2-inch) piece fresh ginger, peeled and cut into
   pieces°°
1 teaspoon soy sauce
1 teaspoon lemon juice
1 pound uncooked large shrimp, cleaned (keep
   tails on)

In food processor or blender, purée all ingredients
except shrimp. In large shallow baking dish, combine
dressing mixture with shrimp. Cover and marinate in
refrigerator, stirring occasionally, at least 3 hours.

Remove shrimp and marinade to large shallow baking
pan or aluminum-foil-lined broiler rack. Broil shrimp
with marinade, turning once, 10 minutes or until
done. Serve remaining marinade with shrimp.
Garnish as desired.

°Substitution: Use ⅓ medium onion, cut into pieces.
°°Substitution: Use 1 teaspoon ground ginger.

Nutrients per serving (1 appetizer):

Calories	24	Sodium	178 mg
Fat	0 g	Cholesterol	23 mg

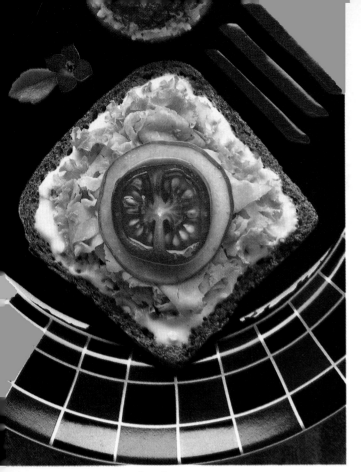

Party Ham Sandwiches

Hot Dog Biscuit Bites

Low Sodium

Makes 40 wedges

¼ cup plain nonfat yogurt
2 tablespoons chopped onion
½ tablespoon prepared mustard
1 (7½-ounce) package refrigerated
    buttermilk biscuits
2 to 3 ARMOUR® Low Fat Lower Salt Jumbo
    Meat Hot Dogs, thinly sliced
3 tablespoons low sodium catsup

Preheat oven to 375°F. Combine yogurt, onion and mustard in small bowl; mix well. Cut each biscuit into 4 wedges. Flatten each wedge out with bottom of a glass. Spread yogurt mixture on wedges; press 1 hot dog slice in center of each. Spray baking sheet with nonstick cooking spray; place wedges on sheet. Bake about 8 to 10 minutes, or until puffy and golden brown. Top with small amount of catsup.

Nutrients per serving (1 wedge):			
Calories	23	Sodium	75 mg
Fat	1 g	Cholesterol	2 mg

Pan Roasted Herbed Almonds

Low Cholesterol

Makes 2 cups

1 teaspoon *each* dried thyme, oregano and basil
½ teaspoon *each* garlic salt and onion powder
¼ teaspoon ground black pepper
2 tablespoons HOLLYWOOD® Peanut Oil
¾ pound (about 2 cups) whole blanched almonds

In a small bowl, combine seasonings. In a large skillet, heat oil over low heat, add almonds and seasonings and cook slowly, stirring, until almonds are lightly browned, approximately 10 minutes. Place mixture on paper towels to absorb excess oil. Can be served immediately or at room temperature.

Note: As almonds cool, seasonings will not adhere, however, herb flavor will remain.

Nutrients per serving (2 tablespoons):			
Calories	122	Sodium	135 mg
Fat	6 g	Cholesterol	0 mg

Party Ham Sandwiches

Quick & Easy

Makes 24 sandwiches

¾ cup plain nonfat yogurt
3 teaspoons chopped fresh chives
1 teaspoon dill mustard
1 loaf party rye or pumpernickel bread
    Leaf lettuce, washed, torn and well drained
1 ARMOUR® Lower Salt Ham Nugget (about
    1¾ pounds), shaved
1 small cucumber, thinly sliced
12 cherry tomatoes, cut in half

Combine yogurt, chives and mustard in small bowl. Arrange bread slices on serving tray; spread evenly with yogurt mixture. Layer lettuce, ham, cucumber slice and tomato half on top of each bread slice. Garnish serving tray with lettuce and green onions, if desired.

Nutrients per serving (1 sandwich):			
Calories	101	Sodium	413 mg
Fat	3 g	Cholesterol	16 mg

Hot Curried V8

Makes 1½ cups or 2 servings

1 teaspoon butter or margarine
¼ cup finely chopped onion
½ teaspoon curry powder
1½ cups V8 vegetable juice *or* no salt added
    V8 vegetable juice
    Alfalfa sprouts for garnish (optional)

1. In 1-quart saucepan over medium-heat, in hot butter, cook onion with curry until onion is tender. Add V8 juice. Heat to boiling.

2. In covered blender or food processor, blend hot mixture until smooth. To serve: Pour into mugs. Garnish with alfalfa sprouts.

Nutrients per serving:			
Calories	62	Sodium	587 mg
Fat	2 g	Cholesterol	6 mg

Sparkling V8

Makes 4¾ cups or 6 servings

3 cups V8 vegetable juice *or* no salt added
    V8 vegetable juice
2 bottles (6½ ounces *each*) sparkling mineral
    water, chilled
    Mint leaves for garnish

1. In small pitcher, mix V8 juice and sparkling mineral water.

2. To serve: Pour over ice cubes in 10-ounce glasses. Garnish with mint leaves.

Nutrients per serving:			
Calories	24	Sodium	378 mg
Fat	0 g	Cholesterol	0 mg

Pineapple Raspberry Punch

Makes 12 servings

5 cups DOLE® Pineapple Juice
1 quart raspberry cranberry drink
1 pint fresh raspberries or frozen raspberries
1 lemon, thinly sliced
    Ice

Chill ingredients. Combine in punch bowl.

Nutrients per serving:			
Calories	121	Sodium	4 mg
Fat	.2 g	Cholesterol	0 mg

Mexicali Sipper

Makes 4½ cups or 6 servings

4 cups V8 vegetable juice *or* no salt added
    V8 vegetable juice
1 canned jalapeño pepper, seeded
2 sprigs fresh cilantro
1 tablespoon lemon juice
1 small ripe avocado, halved, seeded, peeled and
    sliced
    Sweet red pepper rings for garnish
    Green onion brushes for garnish°

1. In covered blender or food processor, blend V8 juice, jalapeño pepper, cilantro, lemon juice and avocado until smooth.

2. To serve: Pour over ice cubes in 10-ounce glasses. Garnish with red pepper rings and green onion brushes.

°Note: To make green onion brushes, slice off the roots and tops of green onions. Leaving at least 3 inches in the center, make lengthwise cuts from center to ends at one or both ends to make a fringe. Place the green onions in a bowl of ice water for a few hours. The ends will curl to look like brushes.

Nutrients per serving:			
Calories	74	Sodium	544 mg
Fat	4 g	Cholesterol	0 mg

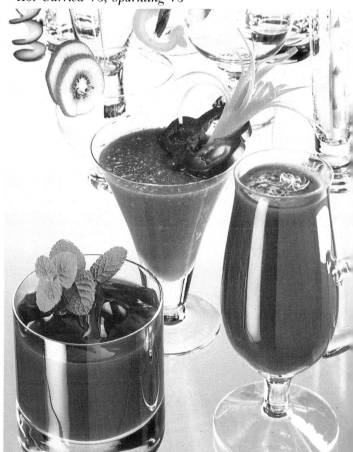

Clockwise from top: Mexicali Sipper, Hot Curried V8, Sparkling V8

Two-Tone Lite Ricotta Loaf

Low Cholesterol

Makes 8 servings

2 envelopes unflavored gelatin
1 cup skim milk

Pepper Layer

1 container (15 ounces) POLLY-O LITE®
    Reduced-Fat Ricotta Cheese
1 jar (7 ounces) roasted red peppers, undrained
¼ teaspoon salt
    Pinch ground pepper

Basil Layer

1 container (15 ounces) POLLY-O LITE®
    Reduced-Fat Ricotta Cheese
1 cup fresh basil leaves
⅓ cup fresh parsley leaves
¾ teaspoon salt
1 small garlic clove, crushed
    Pinch ground pepper
½ cup skim milk
    Additional basil leaves (optional garnish)

In small saucepan, sprinkle gelatin over cold milk; let stand 5 minutes. Stir over low heat until gelatin is completely dissolved.

Pepper Layer: In food processor, puree ricotta with roasted red peppers and their juice, salt and pepper. Add ½ cup dissolved gelatin and process until combined. Pour into an 8×4-inch loaf pan; refrigerate until partially set, about 20 minutes.

Basil Layer: In food processor, combine ricotta, basil, parsley, salt, garlic and pepper. Process until herbs are finely chopped. Add remaining gelatin mixture and skim milk. Pour into a bowl and chill, stirring occasionally, until mixture is consistency of unbeaten egg whites. Spoon over partially set red pepper layer; smooth top. Cover and refrigerate until set, at least 4 hours or overnight. To serve, unmold onto a serving dish. If desired, garnish with fresh basil leaves.

Nutrients per serving:			
Calories	167	Sodium	382 mg
Fat	4 g	Cholesterol	20 mg

Choco-Berry Splash

Quick & Easy

Makes one 12-ounce serving

    Crushed ice
¾ cup skim milk
¼ cup sliced fresh strawberries
2 tablespoons HERSHEY'S® Syrup
2 tablespoons vanilla ice milk
2 tablespoons club soda

Fill tall glass with crushed ice. Measure all ingredients except club soda into blender container. Cover; blend on medium speed until smooth. Pour into glass over crushed ice; add club soda. Serve immediately.

Nutrients per serving:			
Calories	182	Sodium	129 mg
Fat	2 g	Cholesterol	6 mg

Two-Tone Lite Ricotta Loaf

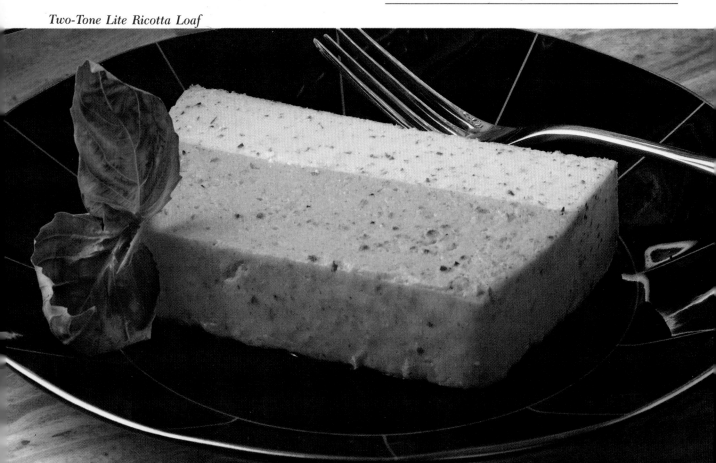

Spicy Chicken Bites

Low Sodium

Makes 4 servings

½ cup lemon juice
¼ cup water
1 tablespoon dried rosemary, crushed
2 cloves garlic, minced
1 teaspoon hot pepper sauce
1 teaspoon Worcestershire sauce
2 boneless, skinless chicken breast halves, cut into small cubes
1 slice mixed grain bread, toasted
¼ cup BLUE DIAMOND® Chopped Natural Almonds, toasted
2 egg whites, lightly beaten

Combine lemon juice, water, rosemary, garlic, hot pepper sauce and Worcestershire sauce in small bowl. Stir in chicken cubes; cover and chill 24 hours. In blender or food processor, process toast to coarse crumbs. Remove to a small bowl; stir in almonds. Lift chicken from marinade. Roll in egg whites, then in crumb mixture to coat evenly. Place on nonstick baking sheet. Bake at 400°F for 10 to 12 minutes. Serve hot or cold.

Nutrients per serving:			
Calories	150	Sodium	100 mg
Fat	5 g	Cholesterol	34 mg

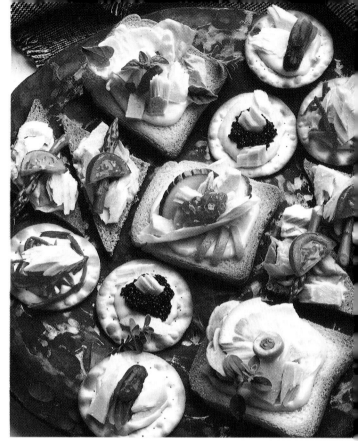

Scandinavian Smörgåsbord

Strawberry Fizz

Quick & Easy

Makes 4 servings

1 can (5 fluid ounces) PET® Evaporated Milk *or* PET® Light Evaporated Skimmed milk
⅔ cup lemon-lime or orange soda, regular or diet
1½ cups fresh *or* frozen strawberries
4 teaspoons sugar or 1 teaspoon artificial sweetener

Combine all ingredients in a blender until smooth. Serve immediately.

Note: Frozen fruit makes the smoothie icy cold; if using fresh fruit, we suggest serving the smoothie over crushed ice.

Nutrients per serving (with PET® Evaporated Milk, regular soda and sugar):			
Calories	99	Sodium	44 mg
Fat	3 g	Cholesterol	10 mg

Nutrients per serving (with PET® Light Evaporated Skimmed milk, diet soda and artificial sweetener):			
Calories	45	Sodium	45 mg
Fat	0 g	Cholesterol	1 mg

Scandinavian Smörgåsbord

Low Sodium

Makes 36 appetizers

36 slices party bread, crackers or flat bread
Reduced-calorie mayonnaise or salad dressing
Mustard
36 small lettuce leaves or Belgian endive leaves
1 can (6½ ounces) STARKIST® Tuna, drained and flaked or broken into chunks
2 hard-cooked eggs, sliced
¼ pound frozen cooked bay shrimp, thawed
½ medium cucumber, thinly sliced
36 pieces steamed asparagus tips or pea pods
Capers, plain yogurt, dill sprigs, pimento strips, red or black caviar, sliced green onion for garnish (optional)

Arrange party bread on a tray; spread each with 1 teaspoon mayonnaise and/or mustard. Top with a small lettuce leaf. Top with tuna, egg slices, shrimp, cucumber or steamed vegetables. Garnish as desired.

Nutrients per serving (1 appetizer):			
Calories	47	Sodium	103 mg
Fat	1 g	Cholesterol	24 mg

Blue Cheese Ball

Low Cholesterol

Makes 1 cheese ball or 24 servings

1 package (8 ounces) cream cheese or reduced-calorie cream cheese, softened
1 package (4 ounces) blue cheese, crumbled
3 tablespoons milk
1 cup chopped pecans, toasted°
 Chopped fresh parsley
 Pecan halves for garnish (optional)

1. In medium bowl with mixer at medium speed, beat cream cheese, blue cheese and milk until smooth and creamy. Stir in chopped pecans. Cover; refrigerate about 2 hours or until firm enough to shape.

2. Shape cheese mixture into ball; roll in chopped parsley to coat. Garnish cheese ball with additional pecan halves, if desired. Serve with crackers and fresh fruit.

°To toast pecans, spread on cookie sheet. Bake, uncovered, at 300°F for 15 minutes or until toasted, stirring once.

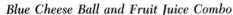

Nutrients per serving (1 tablespoon):			
Calories	81	Sodium	95 mg
Fat	8 g	Cholesterol	14 mg

Favorite Recipe from Wisconsin Milk Marketing Board, Inc.

Blue Cheese Ball and Fruit Juice Combo

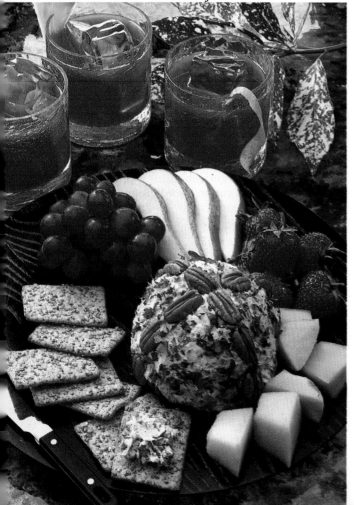

Fruit Juice Combo

Low Sodium

Makes 8 cups or 8 servings

1 cup V8 vegetable juice *or* no salt added
 V8 vegetable juice
1 cup CAMPBELL'S tomato juice
1 cup apple juice
1 cup cranberry juice
1 cup grapefruit juice
1 cup lemonade
1 cup orange juice
1 cup pineapple juice
8 drops hot pepper sauce

In large pitcher, combine all ingredients. To serve: Pour over ice cubes in 10-ounce glasses.

Nutrients per serving:			
Calories	99	Sodium	196 mg
Fat	0 g	Cholesterol	0 mg

Skim Milk Hot Cocoa

Low Sodium

Makes two 7-ounce servings

2 tablespoons HERSHEY'S® Cocoa
3 tablespoons sugar
¼ cup hot water
1½ cups skim milk
⅛ teaspoon vanilla

Blend cocoa and sugar in small saucepan; gradually add hot water. Cook over medium heat, stirring constantly, until mixture boils; boil and stir for 2 minutes. Add milk; heat thoroughly. Stir occasionally; do not boil. Remove from heat; add vanilla. Serve hot.

Nutrients per serving:			
Calories	161	Sodium	97 mg
Fat	1 g	Cholesterol	3 mg

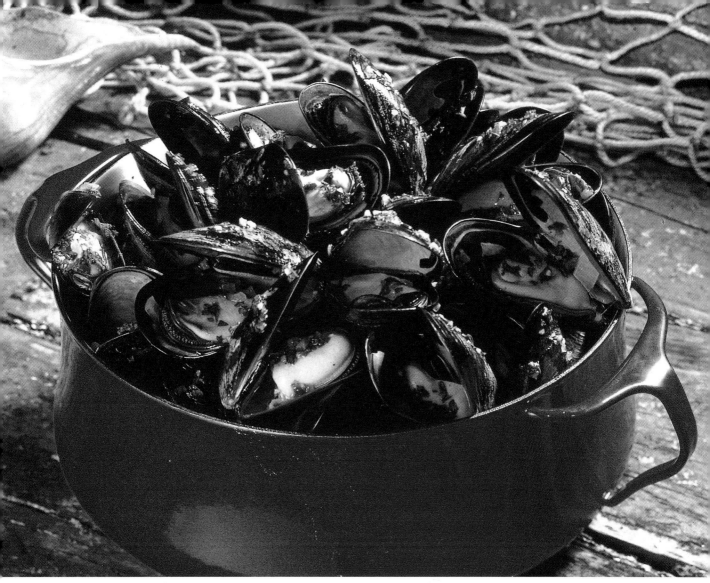

Steamed Mussels in White Wine

Steamed Mussels in White Wine

Low Cholesterol

Makes 6 appetizer servings

⅓ cup Lite WISH-BONE® Italian Dressing
½ cup chopped shallots or onions
3 pounds mussels, well scrubbed
⅔ cup dry white wine
½ cup chopped parsley
¼ cup water
Generous dash crushed red pepper

In large saucepan or stockpot, heat Italian dressing and cook shallots over medium heat, stirring occasionally, 2 minutes or until tender. Add remaining ingredients. Bring to a boil, then simmer covered 4 minutes or until mussel shells open. (Discard any unopened shells.) Serve, if desired, with Italian or French bread.

Nutrients per serving:

Calories	74	Sodium	378 mg
Fat	1 g	Cholesterol	18 mg

Frosty Juice Shake

Low Sodium

Makes 1 serving

1 cup ice cubes
⅔ cup any flavor fruit juice
1 small ripe banana, sliced
⅓ cup QUAKER® Oat Bran hot cereal, uncooked
½ to 1 teaspoon sugar or sugar substitute
(optional)
Dash of cinnamon

Place all ingredients in blender container or food processor bowl; cover. Blend or process on high speed until smooth and thick. Serve immediately.

Nutrients per serving:

Calories	250	Sodium	5 mg
Fat	3 g	Cholesterol	0 mg

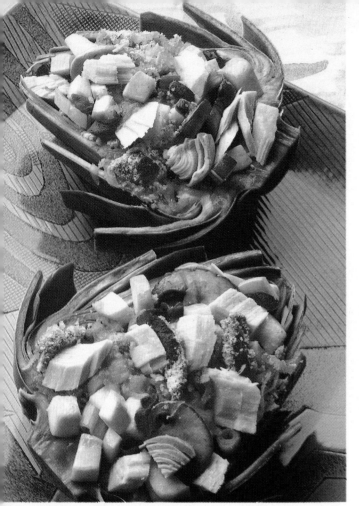

Tuna-Stuffed Artichokes

Low-Calorie Lemonade

Makes about 1 quart

3¼ cups cold water
½ cup REALEMON® Lemon Juice from
    Concentrate
4 to 8 envelopes sugar substitute *or* 1½ teaspoons
    liquid sugar substitute

Combine ingredients; mix well. Serve over ice.
Garnish as desired.

For 1 serving: Combine ¾ cup cold water, 2
tablespoons REALEMON® Brand and 1 to 2
envelopes sugar substitute *or* ½ teaspoon liquid sugar
substitute.

Minted Lemonade: Stir 2 to 3 drops peppermint
extract into 1 quart lemonade.

Sparkling Lemonade: Substitute club soda for cold
water.

Nutrients per serving:

Calories	14	Sodium	9 mg
Fat	0 g	Cholesterol	0 mg

Tuna-Stuffed Artichokes

Low Cholesterol

Makes 8 appetizer servings

4 medium artichokes
    Lemon juice
1½ cups chopped fresh mushrooms
1 cup diced yellow squash or zucchini
⅓ cup chopped green onions
1 clove garlic, minced
2 tablespoons vegetable oil
1 can (12½ ounces) STARKIST® Tuna, drained
    and flaked
½ cup shredded low-fat Cheddar, mozzarella or
    Monterey Jack cheese
¼ cup seasoned bread crumbs
2 tablespoons diced drained pimento

With a kitchen shear trim sharp points from artichoke
leaves. Trim stems; remove loose outer leaves. Cut 1
inch from the tops. Brush cut edges with lemon juice.
In a large covered saucepan or Dutch oven bring
artichokes and salted water to a boil; reduce heat.
Simmer until a leaf pulls out easily, 20 to 30 minutes.
Drain upside down.

Preheat oven to 450°F. When cool enough to handle,
cut artichokes lengthwise into halves. Remove fuzzy
chokes and hearts. Finely chop hearts; discard chokes.
In a medium skillet sauté mushrooms, artichoke
hearts, squash, onions and garlic in oil for 3 minutes,
stirring frequently. Stir in tuna. Place artichoke
halves, cut side up, in a lightly oiled baking dish.
Mound tuna mixture in center of artichokes. In a
small bowl stir together cheese, bread crumbs and
pimento; sprinkle over filling. Bake for 5 to 8
minutes, or until cheese is melted and topping is
golden.

Nutrients per serving:

Calories	136	Sodium	522 mg
Fat	10 g	Cholesterol	47 mg

Chocolate Egg Cream

Low Cholesterol

Makes 3 (8-ounce) servings

1 envelope KNOX® Unflavored Gelatine
1¼ cups cold skim or whole milk
¼ cup chocolate syrup
2 tablespoons sugar
1 cup ice cubes (6 to 8)
    Cola, club soda or seltzer

In small saucepan, sprinkle unflavored gelatine over
¼ cup cold milk; let stand 1 minute. Stir over low
heat until gelatine is completely dissolved, about 4
minutes.

In blender, process remaining 1 cup milk, syrup and sugar. While processing, through feed cap, gradually add gelatine mixture and process until blended. Add ice cubes, 1 at a time; process at high speed until ice is melted. Pour into glasses and top with a splash of cola.

Hint: To make ahead: After ice is melted, chill blender container. To serve: Process in blender.

Nutrients per serving:			
Calories	149	Sodium	67 mg
Fat	1 g	Cholesterol	4 mg

Christmas Punch

Low Sodium

Makes 12 servings

5 cups DOLE® Pineapple Juice
1 bottle (24 ounces) sparkling apple juice or champagne

Chill punch ingredients. Combine in punch bowl. Float ice mold in punch when ready to serve.

Ice Mold:

1 can (20 ounces) DOLE® Pineapple Chunks
1 orange, sliced, quartered
1 pint strawberries
Mint sprigs

Combine undrained pineapple, fruit and mint in 6-cup mold. Add enough water or juice to fill. Freeze.

Nutrients per serving:			
Calories	132	Sodium	4 mg
Fat	0 g	Cholesterol	0 mg

Cooler-Than-Cool Yogurt Drink

Quick & Easy

Makes 4 servings

2 cups plain lowfat yogurt
1 small ripe avocado, diced
⅔ cup cubed, seeded, pared cucumber
5 or 6 fresh mint leaves *or* ½ teaspoon dried mint leaves
½ teaspoon celery salt
¼ teaspoon TABASCO® pepper sauce
1 cup cracked ice
Additional mint leaves for garnish (optional)

In blender combine all ingredients except garnish. Cover. Process until smooth. Garnish with fresh mint, if desired.

Nutrients per serving:			
Calories	160	Sodium	310 mg
Fat	10 g	Cholesterol	10 mg

Italian Bread Pizza

Quick & Easy

Makes 12 appetizer servings

1 large loaf Italian bread
1½ cups (6 ounces) shredded ARMOUR® Lower Salt Monterey Jack Cheese, divided
1 (16-ounce) jar prepared no salt added, no sugar, no fat pasta sauce
1½ tablespoons dried Italian seasoning
12 ounces ARMOUR® Lower Salt Ham, thinly sliced
1 (20-ounce) can pineapple rings, well drained
8 thin green pepper rings
8 thin red pepper rings

Slice bread lengthwise in half. Toast cut sides under broiler until lightly browned. Sprinkle ¼ cup of the cheese on each half; broil again about 1 to 2 minutes, or until cheese is melted. Combine pasta sauce and seasoning in small saucepan; cook over medium heat until hot. Spoon sauce evenly over bread halves, top evenly with ham and pineapple rings. Place green and red pepper rings alternately on top. Sprinkle each half with ½ cup of remaining cheese; place on baking sheet. Broil 4 to 5 inches from heat source about 4 to 6 minutes, or until cheese is melted. Cut each half into 6 pieces. Garnish with parsley, if desired.

Nutrients per serving:			
Calories	253	Sodium	482 mg
Fat	6 g	Cholesterol	29 mg

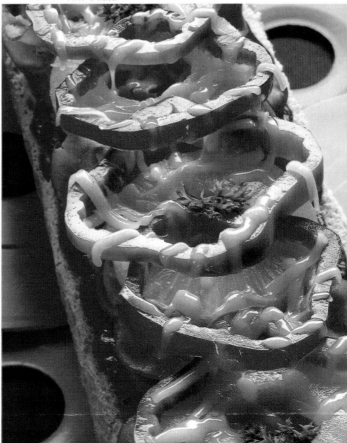

Italian Bread Pizza

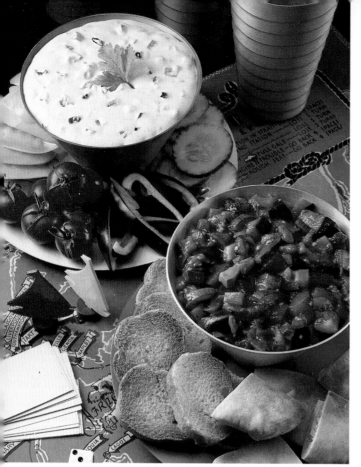

Creamy Chili Dip and Ratatouille Appetizer

Creamy Chili Dip

Low Sodium

Makes 4 cups

2 packages (8 ounces *each*) cream cheese or
   reduced-calorie cream cheese, softened
¾ cup V8 vegetable juice
1 can (4 ounces) chopped green chilies
½ cup chopped pitted ripe olives
½ cup chopped sweet red pepper
2 teaspoons grated onion
¼ teaspoon hot pepper sauce
   Fresh cilantro for garnish
   Fresh vegetables or chips

1. In medium bowl with mixer at medium speed, beat cream cheese until smooth and fluffy.

2. Gradually beat in V8 juice until smooth and thoroughly blended.

3. Stir in chilies, olives, red pepper, onion and hot pepper sauce. Cover; refrigerate until serving time, at least 4 hours.

4. Garnish with fresh cilantro. Serve with fresh vegetables or chips for dipping.

Nutrients per serving (1 tablespoon):			
Calories	27	Sodium	50 mg
Fat	3 g	Cholesterol	8 mg

Ratatouille Appetizer

Low Cholesterol

¼ cup olive oil
1 large onion, chopped
2 cloves garlic, minced
1 teaspoon dried Italian seasoning, crushed
1 small eggplant, cut into ¼-inch cubes
   (about ¾ pound)
1 large sweet red pepper, cut into ¼-inch pieces
1 small zucchini, cut into ¼-inch cubes
¾ cup V8 vegetable juice
   Toasted French bread or pita bread wedges

1. In 4-quart saucepan over medium heat, in hot oil, cook onion with garlic and Italian seasoning until onion is tender, stirring often. Stir in eggplant, red pepper and zucchini. Cook 10 minutes or until eggplant is tender, stirring often.

2. Stir in V8 juice; cook 3 minutes. Serve warm or chilled, with toasted French bread or pita bread wedges.

Nutrients per serving (1 tablespoon):			
Calories	13	Sodium	11 mg
Fat	1 g	Cholesterol	0 mg

Confetti Tuna in Celery Sticks

Low Sodium

Makes 10 pieces

1 can (3¼ ounces) STARKIST® Tuna, drained and
   flaked
½ cup shredded red or green cabbage
½ cup shredded carrot
¼ cup shredded yellow squash or zucchini
3 tablespoons reduced-calorie cream cheese,
   softened
1 tablespoon plain low-fat yogurt
½ teaspoon dried basil, crushed
   Salt and pepper to taste
10 to 12 (4-inch) celery sticks with leaves, if
   desired

In a small bowl toss together tuna, cabbage, carrot and squash. Stir in cream cheese, yogurt and basil. Add salt and pepper to taste. With small spatula spread mixture into celery sticks.

Nutrients per serving (1 piece):			
Calories	32	Sodium	92 mg
Fat	2 g	Cholesterol	9 mg

Grilled Mushrooms with Lamb and Herbs

Makes 6 servings

¼ cup olive oil
¼ cup fresh lime juice
 1 small green onion, minced
½ teaspoon fresh ginger, grated
¼ teaspoon salt
¼ teaspoon black pepper
 1 bunch parsley
 6 ounces cooked American lamb°, cut in ½-inch
    cubes or to fit mushroom caps
36 medium mushroom caps

Combine all ingredients except lamb and mushrooms
in blender and process until finely minced. Brush
each mushroom generously with mixture and arrange
on baking sheet. Top each mushroom with a lamb
cube. Broil about 4 inches from heat source until hot.
Garnish with parsley, if desired.

°Leftover leg of lamb may be used.

Nutrients per serving:

Calories	62	Sodium	14 mg
Fat	4 g	Cholesterol	20 mg

Favorite recipe from **American Lamb Council**

Pineapple Shrimp Appetizers

Makes 30 appetizers

1 can (8 ounces) DOLE® Crushed Pineapple,
   drained
1 can (4¼ ounces) Pacific shrimp, drained
¼ cup reduced calorie mayonnaise
1 tablespoon minced green onion
2 teaspoons Dijon-style mustard
½ teaspoon dill weed
2 cucumbers

Combine all ingredients except cucumbers. Cut
cucumbers in ⅛ to ¼-inch thick slices. Spoon heaping
teaspoon of pineapple mixture on top of each slice.
Garnish with dill or minced green onion if desired.

*Variation: Omit mustard and dill weed. Add 2
teaspoons minced cilantro and dash of cayenne
pepper.*

Nutrients per serving (1 appetizer):

Calories	15	Sodium	15 mg
Fat	0g	Cholesterol	6 mg

Grilled Mushrooms with Lamb and Herbs

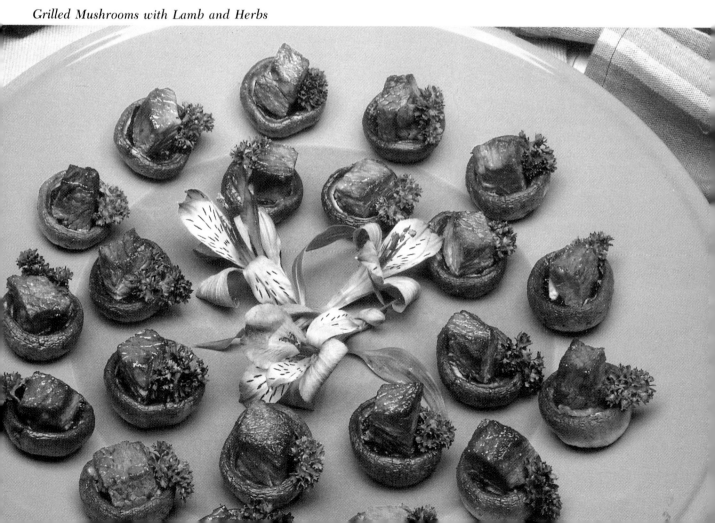

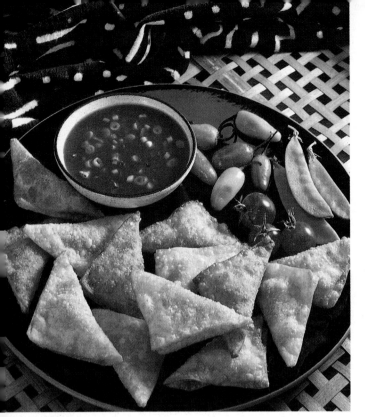

Chili-Cheese Wontons with Cilantro Sauce

Garden Vegetable Dip

> **Low Sodium**

Makes 5½ cups dip

1 bunch DOLE® Broccoli
1 head DOLE® Cauliflower
1 pound DOLE® Carrots
½ cup minced onion
2 packages (8 ounces *each*) cream cheese,
   softened
1 teaspoon dill weed
½ teaspoon ground cumin
¼ teaspoon chili powder
⅛ teaspoon salt
10 drops hot pepper sauce
   Vegetable dippers:
      broccoli and cauliflower flowerets, carrots,
      celery, cucumber slices, bell pepper strips,
      mushroom slices, cherry tomatoes

Break broccoli and cauliflower into flowerets. Mince 1 cup of each, reserve remaining flowerets for vegetable dippers. Mince 1 cup of carrots, slice remaining for dippers. In food processor fitted with metal blade, combine minced broccoli, cauliflower, carrots, onion, cream cheese and seasonings; process until smooth. Refrigerate 3 hours, or overnight, in covered serving bowl. Serve with vegetable dippers and crackers.

Nutrients per serving (1 tablespoon of dip):			
Calories	19	Sodium	19 mg
Fat	2 g	Cholesterol	6 mg

Chili-Cheese Wontons with Cilantro Sauce

> **Low Cholesterol**

Makes 25 appetizers

¾ cup V8 vegetable juice
2 tablespoons chopped fresh cilantro or parsley
2 tablespoons chopped green onion
1 tablespoon vegetable oil
½ cup chopped onion
⅓ cup chopped sweet red pepper
2 teaspoons chili powder
1 can (4 ounces) chopped green chilies
1 cup shredded Monterey Jack cheese (4 ounces)
25 wonton wrappers
   Oil for deep-fat frying

1. To make sauce: In small bowl, stir together V8 juice, cilantro and green onion; set aside.

2. To make filling: In 8-inch skillet over medium heat, in 1 tablespoon hot oil, cook onion and red pepper with chili powder until onion is tender, stirring occasionally. Remove from heat; cool slightly. Stir in chilies and cheese.

3. Keep wonton wrappers covered with plastic wrap until ready to fill. Spoon about 1½ teaspoons filling in center of each wonton wrapper. Moisten edges with water; fold diagonally in half. Pinch edges to seal. Cover filled wontons with plastic wrap while working with remaining wonton wrappers.

4. In large saucepan over medium-high heat, heat 1½ inches oil to 350°F. Adjust heat to maintain temperature. Cook wontons, 4 at a time, 1 to 2 minutes or until golden brown on both sides. Remove to paper towels to drain.

5. Serve warm with sauce for dipping.

Note: Fried wontons can be frozen. To reheat, preheat oven to 350°F. Place wontons on cookie sheet; bake 15 minutes or until crisp.

Nutrients per serving (1 appetizer):			
Calories	54	Sodium	79 mg
Fat	3 g	Cholesterol	4 mg

Lemony Fruit Dip

> **Quick & Easy**

½ cup MIRACLE WHIP® Cholesterol Free
   Dressing
½ cup lowfat lemon flavored yogurt

Combine ingredients; mix well. Chill. Serve with fruit.

Nutrients per serving (1 tablespoon):			
Calories	80	Sodium	90 mg
Fat	7 g	Cholesterol	0 mg

Eggplant Caviar

Makes 1½ cups

1 large eggplant, unpeeled
¼ cup chopped onion
2 tablespoons lemon juice
1 tablespoon olive or vegetable oil
1 small clove garlic
½ teaspoon salt
¼ teaspoon TABASCO® pepper sauce
   Cooked egg white, sieved (optional)
   Lemon slice (optional)

Preheat oven to 350°F. Pierce eggplant with fork. Place eggplant in shallow baking dish. Bake 1 hour or until soft, turning once. Trim off ends; slice eggplant in half lengthwise. Place cut-side-down in colander and let drain 10 minutes. Scoop out pulp; reserve pulp and peel. In blender or food processor combine eggplant peel, onion, lemon juice, oil, garlic, salt and TABASCO® sauce. Cover; process until peel is finely chopped. Add eggplant pulp. Cover; process just until chopped. Place in serving dish. Garnish with egg white and lemon slice, if desired. Serve with toast points.

Nutrients per serving (1 tablespoon):

Calories	10	Sodium	45 mg
Fat	1 g	Cholesterol	0 mg

Imperial Pineapple Nog

Makes 8 servings

6 cups DOLE® Pineapple Juice
   Peel from 1 orange°
½ teaspoon ground cinnamon
¼ teaspoon ground nutmeg
1 carton (4 ounces) frozen whipped topping, thawed
½ cup honey

Combine pineapple juice, orange peel, cinnamon and nutmeg in Dutch oven. Heat just to boil. Remove from heat. Add topping and honey. Whisk into hot pineapple juice mixture. Sprinkle servings with additional nutmeg and cinnamon if desired.

°*Spiral cut peel from orange with vegetable peeler.*

Nutrients per serving:

Calories	184	Sodium	4 mg
Fat	1 g	Cholesterol	0 mg

Frosty Chocolate Shake

Makes 2 servings

1 teaspoon KNOX® Unflavored Gelatine
½ cup skim milk
2 tablespoons chocolate syrup
2 packets aspartame sweetener
¼ teaspoon vanilla extract
1 cup ice cubes (6 to 8)

In small saucepan, sprinkle unflavored gelatine over ¼ cup milk; let stand 1 minute. Stir over low heat until gelatine is completely dissolved, about 5 minutes.

In blender, process remaining ¼ cup milk, syrup, sweetener and vanilla until blended. While processing, through feed cap, gradually add gelatine mixture and process until blended. Add ice cubes, 1 at a time; process at high speed until ice is melted.

Nutrients per serving:

Calories	77	Sodium	45 mg
Fat	1 g	Cholesterol	3 mg

Frosty Chocolate Shake

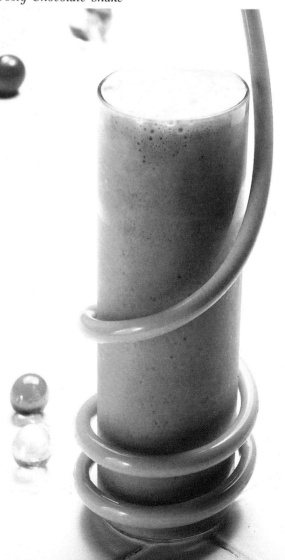

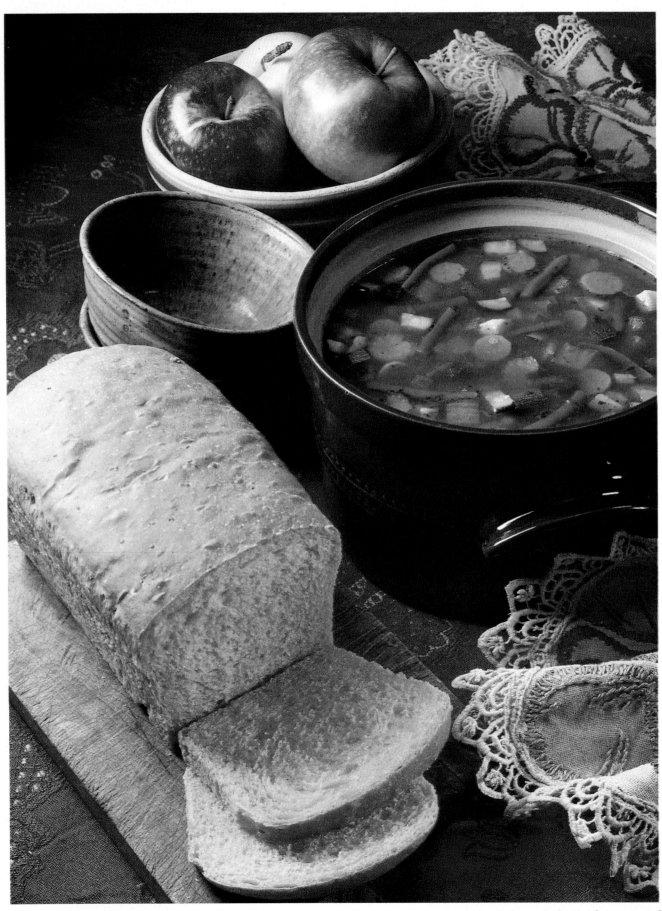

Harvest Bowl Soup and V8 Cheese Bread

Soups & Breads

Harvest Bowl Soup

Low Cholesterol

Makes 14 cups or 14 side-dish servings

1 tablespoon olive oil
2 cups chopped onions
1½ cups thinly sliced carrots
1 cup thinly sliced celery
4 cloves garlic, minced
2 teaspoons dried Italian seasoning, crushed
3 cans (14½ ounces *each*) SWANSON clear ready to serve chicken broth or 4 cans (10½ ounces *each*) CAMPBELL'S ready to serve low sodium chicken broth
3 cups V8 vegetable juice or no salt added V8 vegetable juice
¼ pound green beans, cut into pieces
1 bay leaf
⅛ teaspoon pepper
2 cans (16 ounces *each*) red or white kidney beans, drained
2 cups coarsely chopped zucchini or yellow squash

1. In 6-quart Dutch oven over medium heat, in hot oil, cook onions, carrots and celery with garlic and Italian seasoning until vegetables are tender, stirring often.

2. Stir in remaining ingredients, except kidney beans and zucchini. Heat to boiling; reduce heat to low. Cover; simmer 30 minutes.

3. Stir in kidney beans and zucchini. Cover; simmer 5 minutes or until zucchini is tender. Discard bay leaf.

Note: When using low sodium chicken broth and no salt added V8 juice for the soup, add 1 tablespoon lemon juice with the kidney beans and zucchini.

Nutrients per serving:

Calories	94	Sodium	706 mg
Fat	2 g	Cholesterol	0 mg

V8 Cheese Bread

Low Cholesterol

Makes 2 loaves, 12 slices each

5½ to 6 cups all-purpose flour, divided
2 packages active dry yeast
1½ teaspoons salt
1 cup V8 vegetable juice
¾ cup water
3 tablespoons butter or margarine
1½ cups shredded Cheddar cheese (6 ounces)
1 egg

1. In large bowl, combine 2 cups of the flour, yeast and salt; set aside. In small saucepan over medium heat, heat V8 juice, water and butter until warm (115° to 120°F.).

2. Stir V8 mixture into flour mixture. With mixer at low speed, beat 30 seconds. Add cheese and egg. With mixer at high speed, beat 3 minutes. Stir in 2½ cups of the remaining flour.

3. Turn dough onto lightly floured surface; knead until smooth and elastic, about 6 minutes, adding remaining flour while kneading. Shape dough into ball; place in large greased bowl, turning dough to grease top. Cover; let rise in warm place until doubled in bulk, about 1 hour.

4. Spray two 8- by 4-inch loaf pans with vegetable cooking spray. Punch dough down; divide in half. Shape into 2 loaves. Place in pans. Cover; let rise in warm place until doubled, about 45 minutes.

5. Preheat oven to 375°F. Bake 35 minutes or until golden and loaves sound hollow when lightly tapped with fingers. Remove from pans; cool on wire racks.

Nutrients per serving (1 slice):

Calories	157	Sodium	231 mg
Fat	4 g	Cholesterol	20 mg

Cranberry Oat Bran Muffins

Low Cholesterol

Makes 1 dozen

2 cups flour
1 cup oat bran
½ cup packed brown sugar
2 teaspoons baking powder
½ teaspoon baking soda
½ teaspoon salt (optional)
½ cup MIRACLE WHIP® Cholesterol Free
   Dressing
3 egg whites, slightly beaten
½ cup skim milk
⅓ cup orange juice
1 teaspoon grated orange rind
1 cup coarsely chopped cranberries

Preheat oven to 375°. Line 12 medium muffin cups
with paper baking cups or spray with vegetable
cooking spray. Mix together dry ingredients. Add
combined dressing, egg whites, milk, juice and rind;
mixing just until moistened. Fold in cranberries. Fill
prepared muffin cups almost full. Bake 15 to 17
minutes or until golden brown.

Nutrients per serving (1 muffin):			
Calories	190	Sodium	180 mg
Fat	5 g	Cholesterol	0 mg

Cranberry Oat Bran Muffins

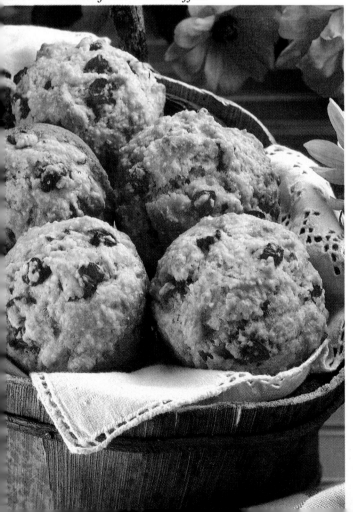

Seafood Gumbo

Makes about 3½ quarts; 12 servings

1 tablespoon reduced calorie margarine
2 cups onions, chopped, in all
1¼ ounces tasso (preferred) or lean ham, minced
1½ cups celery, chopped, in all
1¼ cups bell pepper, chopped, in all
4 cups sliced okra, in all
2 cups peeled and chopped tomatoes
1 tablespoon plus 1 teaspoon Chef Paul
   Prudhomme's SEAFOOD MAGIC®, in all
3 bay leaves
7 cups shrimp stock or water, in all
1 cup oyster liquid°
1½ teaspoons minced garlic, in all
1 teaspoon salt
1 pound peeled shrimp
¼ cup minced green onions (green part only)
1 dozen large *or* 2 dozen medium oysters
½ pound crabmeat, picked over
6 cups hot, cooked rice

Place margarine in a large pot or kettle over high
heat. Add 1 cup chopped onions and the tasso; cook
over high heat, stirring occasionally and scraping the
bottom of the pot with a wooden spoon, about 3½
minutes. Add 1 cup celery and ¾ cup bell pepper.
Lower heat to medium, cover and cook about 2
minutes. Remove cover. Add 3 cups okra and all of
the tomatoes. Mix thoroughly, add 1 tablespoon of the
SEAFOOD MAGIC® and stir, scraping up all the
caramelized browned bits on the bottom of the pot. If
this browned part does not come up easily, add 2
tablespoons of stock and scrape it up. Add the bay
leaves. Cook, covered, over high heat, occasionally
stirring and scraping, about 8 minutes. Stir in 1 cup of
shrimp stock, scrape the bottom of the pot, cover and
cook 12 minutes. Add the oyster liquid, and ½
teaspoon garlic. Stir, using the liquid to help scrape
the bottom of the pot. Cover and cook 11 minutes.
Add 4 cups stock, remaining 1 cup onions, ½ cup
celery, 1 cup okra, ½ cup bell pepper and the
remaining teaspoon of minced garlic. Cook, stirring, 2
minutes. Add 2 more cups of stock and cook another
3 minutes. Stir in the remaining teaspoon of
SEAFOOD MAGIC® and continue cooking for 8
minutes. Add the salt, cook 2 minutes, then stir in the
shrimp, green onions, oysters and crabmeat. Bring to
a boil over high heat, then turn off heat and let it sit 5
to 10 minutes to allow the flavors to develop. Remove
bay leaves before serving.

Serve 1 cup of gumbo over ½ cup rice in each bowl.

*°If there is no liquid with your oysters, or not enough,
you can substitute either stock or water.*

Nutrients per serving (including rice):			
Calories	288	Sodium	1719 mg
Fat	5 g	Cholesterol	108 mg

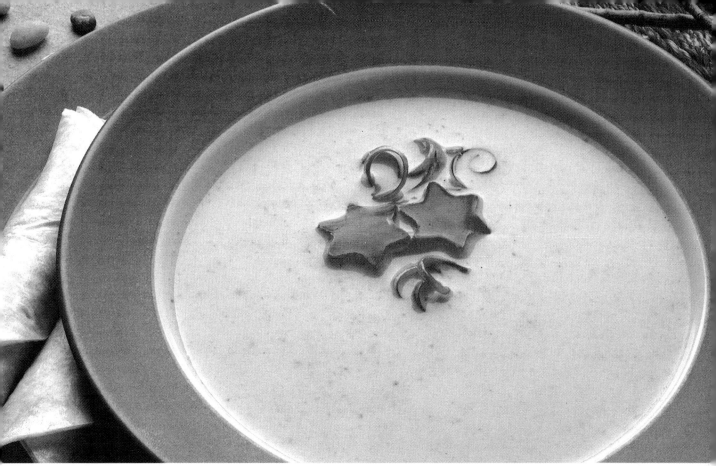

Chicken Cilantro Bisque

Chicken Cilantro Bisque

Quick & Easy

Makes about 4 servings

6 ounces boneless, skinless chicken breasts, cut
 into chunks
2½ cups low-sodium chicken broth
½ cup cilantro leaves
½ cup sliced green onions
¼ cup sliced celery
1 large clove garlic, minced
½ teaspoon ground cumin
⅓ cup all-purpose flour
1½ cups (12-ounce can) *undiluted* CARNATION®
 Evaporated Skimmed Milk
 Fresh ground pepper, to taste

In large saucepan, combine chicken, broth, cilantro, green onions, celery, garlic and cumin. Heat to boiling; reduce heat and boil gently, covered, for 15 minutes. Pour soup into blender container. Add flour. Cover and blend, starting at low speed, until smooth. Pour mixture back into saucepan. Cook over medium heat, stirring constantly, until mixture comes to a boil and thickens. Remove from heat. Gradually stir in milk. Reheat just to serving temperature. Do not boil. Season with pepper to taste. Garnish as desired.

Nutrients per serving:			
Calories	176	Sodium	608 mg
Fat	2 g	Cholesterol	28 mg

Chilled Carrot Soup

Low Cholesterol

Makes 8 servings

2 tablespoons vegetable oil
1 large onion, chopped
1½ teaspoons curry powder
3½ cups chicken broth
1 pound carrots, sliced
2 stalks celery, sliced
1 bay leaf
½ teaspoon ground cumin
½ teaspoon TABASCO® pepper sauce
1 cup milk
1 cup cottage cheese

In large saucepan heat oil; cook onion and curry 3 to 5 minutes. Add broth, carrots, celery, bay leaf, cumin and TABASCO® pepper sauce; mix well. Cover; simmer 25 minutes or until vegetables are tender. Remove bay leaf. Spoon about ⅓ of the carrot mixture, milk and cottage cheese into container of blender or food processor. Cover; process until smooth. Pour into serving bowl. Repeat with remaining mixture, milk and cottage cheese. Cover; refrigerate until chilled. Serve with additional TABASCO® pepper sauce, if desired.

Nutrients per serving:			
Calories	120	Sodium	500 mg
Fat	5 g	Cholesterol	5 mg

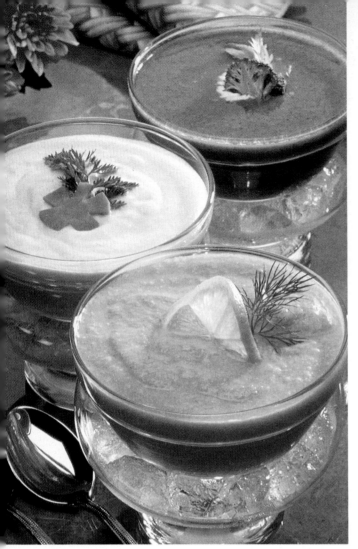

Broccoli Tarragon Soup, Garden Potato Soup and Carrot Lemon Soup

Garden Potato Soup

Quick & Easy

Makes 6 servings

6 cups chicken broth
1 pound potatoes, diced
1 large onion, sliced
½ cup diced DOLE® Celery
½ cup diced DOLE® Carrots
1 bay leaf
¼ teaspoon fines herbes or thyme
¼ cup whipping cream

Combine chicken broth, potatoes, onion, celery, carrots, bay leaf and fines herbes in large saucepan. Bring to boil. Simmer until vegetables are tender, 10 to 15 minutes. Cool. Remove bay leaf. Purée in food processor or blender. Stir in cream. Chill before serving.

Nutrients per serving:

Calories	254	Sodium	796 mg
Fat	5 g	Cholesterol	15 mg

Carrot Lemon Soup

Quick & Easy

Makes 2 servings

1 cup diced DOLE® Carrots
1 can (14½ ounces) chicken broth
1 tablespoon lemon juice
¼ teaspoon grated lemon peel
1 teaspoon sugar
¼ cup half-and-half

Combine carrots, chicken broth, lemon juice, lemon peel and sugar in saucepan. Cook until carrots are tender, 10 to 12 minutes. Purée in blender. Stir in half-and-half.

Nutrients per serving:

Calories	219	Sodium	735 mg
Fat	5 g	Cholesterol	12 mg

Broccoli Tarragon Soup

Low Cholesterol

Makes 2 servings

2 cups DOLE® Broccoli flowerets
1 can (14½ ounces) chicken broth
½ cup chopped onion
¼ teaspoon dried tarragon, crumbled

Combine all ingredients in saucepan. Cook, covered, until broccoli is tender but still bright green. Purée in blender. Chill before serving.

Nutrients per serving:

Calories	184	Sodium	728 mg
Fat	2 g	Cholesterol	1 mg

Touch of Honey Bread

Low Sodium

Makes 16 servings

- 2½ to 3 cups all-purpose flour
- 1 cup QUAKER® Oat Bran hot cereal, uncooked
- 1 package quick-rise yeast
- ½ teaspoon salt
- 1¼ cups water
- 2 tablespoons honey
- 2 tablespoons margarine

In large mixer bowl, combine 1 cup flour, oat bran, yeast and salt. Heat water, honey and margarine until very warm (120° to 130°F). Add to dry ingredients; beat at low speed of electric mixer until moistened. Increase speed to medium; continue beating 3 minutes. Stir in enough remaining flour to form a stiff dough. Lightly spray bowl with vegetable oil cooking spray or oil lightly. Turn dough out onto lightly floured surface. Knead 8 to 10 minutes or until dough is smooth and elastic. Place into prepared bowl, turning once to coat surface of dough. Cover; let rise in warm place 30 minutes or until doubled in size. Lightly spray 8×4-inch loaf pan with vegetable oil cooking spray or oil lightly. Punch down dough. Roll into 15×7-inch rectangle. Starting at narrow end, roll up dough tightly. Pinch ends and seam to seal; place seam side down in prepared pan. Cover; let rise in warm place 30 minutes or until doubled in size. Heat oven to 375°F. Bake 35 to 40 minutes or until golden brown. Remove from pan; cool on wire rack at least 1 hour before slicing.

Nutrients per serving (1 slice):

Calories	120	Sodium	85 mg
Fat	2 g	Cholesterol	0 mg

Whole Wheat Biscuits

Low Cholesterol

Makes 8 biscuits

- 1 cup all-purpose flour
- ½ cup whole wheat flour
- 2 tablespoons sugar
- 2½ teaspoons baking powder
- ½ teaspoon salt (optional)
- 2 tablespoons plus 1½ teaspoons CRISCO® Shortening
- ½ cup skim milk

1. Heat oven to 400°F.

2. Combine all-purpose flour, whole wheat flour, sugar, baking powder and salt (if used) in medium bowl. Mix well. Cut in CRISCO® with pastry blender (or 2 knives) to form coarse crumbs.

3. Add milk. Stir until dry ingredients are just moistened. Place on floured surface. Knead gently with fingertips 8 to 10 times. Pat or roll into 8½-inch circle about ½-inch thick°.

4. With 2½-inch round biscuit cutter, cut 6 biscuits. Press dough scraps into ball and flatten again. Cut 2 biscuits. Place on ungreased baking sheet.

5. Bake at 400°F for 12 to 15 minutes or until golden brown. Serve warm.

°Hint: Cover dough with waxed paper. Press and flatten with 8- or 9-inch round cake pan until dough is desired thickness.

Nutrients per serving (1 biscuit):

Calories	130	Sodium	145 mg
Fat	4 g	Cholesterol	0 mg

Touch of Honey Bread

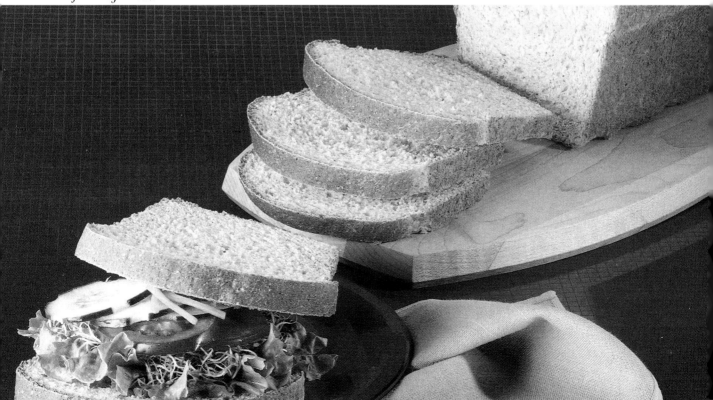

West Coast Bouillabaisse

Quick & Easy

Makes 6 servings

1 cup sliced onions
2 stalks celery, cut diagonally into slices
2 cloves garlic, minced
1 tablespoon vegetable oil
4 cups chicken broth
1 can (28 ounces) tomatoes with juice, cut up
1 can (6½ ounces) minced clams with juice
½ cup dry white wine
1 teaspoon Worcestershire sauce
½ teaspoon dried thyme, crushed
¼ teaspoon bottled hot pepper sauce
1 bay leaf
1 cup frozen cooked bay shrimp, thawed
1 can (6½ ounces) STARKIST® Tuna, drained and broken into chunks
   Salt and pepper to taste
6 slices lemon
6 slices French bread

In a Dutch oven sauté onions, celery and garlic in oil for 3 minutes. Stir in broth, tomatoes with juice, clams with juice, wine, Worcestershire, thyme, hot pepper sauce and bay leaf. Bring to a boil; reduce heat. Simmer for 15 minutes. Stir in shrimp and tuna; cook for 2 minutes to heat. Remove bay leaf. Season with salt and pepper. Garnish with lemon slices and serve with bread.

Nutrients per serving:			
Calories	212	Sodium	1146 mg
Fat	6 g	Cholesterol	70 mg

West Coast Bouillabaisse

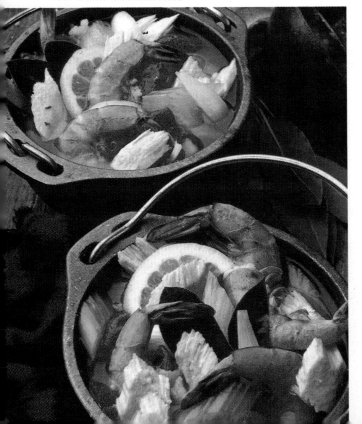

Apricot Muffins

Low Cholesterol

Makes 12 muffins

1¾ cups all-purpose flour
⅓ cup sugar
¼ teaspoon salt (optional)
1 tablespoon baking powder
2 cups KELLOGG'S® COMMON SENSE® Oat Bran cereal, any variety
1½ cups apricot nectar
2 egg whites
¼ cup vegetable oil
½ cup chopped, dried apricots

1. Stir together flour, sugar, salt and baking powder; set aside.

2. In large mixing bowl, combine KELLOGG'S® COMMON SENSE® Oat Bran cereal, apricot nectar, egg whites and oil until thoroughly mixed. Stir in apricots. Add flour mixture, stirring only until combined. Portion batter evenly into 12 lightly greased 2½-inch muffin-pan cups.

3. Bake in 400°F oven about 25 minutes or until golden brown. Serve warm.

Nutrients per serving:			
Calories	200	Sodium	224 mg
Fat	5 g	Cholesterol	0 mg

Turkey Wild Rice Pumpkin Soup

Quick & Easy

Makes 8 servings

2 tablespoons margarine or butter
½ cup chopped onions
½ cup sliced celery
4 cups chicken or turkey broth
1 can (16 ounces) solid-pack pumpkin
2 cups (10 ounces) cubed cooked BUTTERBALL® turkey
2 cups cooked wild rice
1 cup half and half
1 teaspoon seasoned salt
½ teaspoon ground cinnamon

Cook and stir margarine, onions and celery in Dutch oven over medium heat until vegetables are crisp-tender, about 5 minutes. Add broth and pumpkin. Bring to a boil; reduce heat and simmer 5 minutes. Stir in turkey, rice, half and half, salt and cinnamon. Heat to serving temperature; do not boil.

Nutrients per serving:			
Calories	296	Sodium	736 mg
Fat	8 g	Cholesterol	38 mg

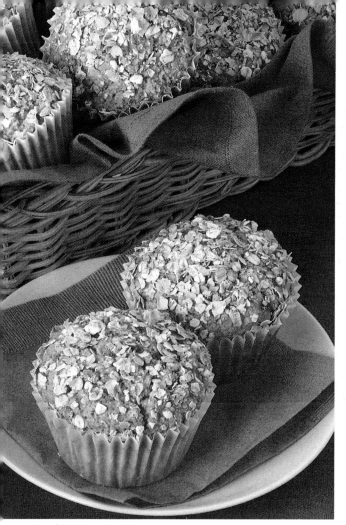

Double Oat Muffins

Double Oat Muffins

Low Sodium

Makes 12 servings

2 cups QUAKER® Oat Bran hot cereal, uncooked
⅓ cup firmly packed brown sugar
¼ cup all-purpose flour
2 teaspoons baking powder
¼ teaspoon salt (optional)
¼ teaspoon nutmeg (optional)
1 cup skim milk
2 egg whites, slightly beaten
3 tablespoons vegetable oil
1½ teaspoons vanilla
¼ cup QUAKER OATS® (quick or old fashioned, uncooked)
1 tablespoon firmly packed brown sugar

Heat oven to 400°F. Line 12 medium muffin cups with paper baking cups. Combine oat bran, ⅓ cup brown sugar, flour, baking powder, salt and nutmeg. Add combined milk, egg whites, oil and vanilla, mixing just until moistened. Fill muffin cups almost full. Combine oats and remaining 1 tablespoon brown sugar; sprinkle evenly over batter. Bake 20 to 22 minutes or until golden brown.

Microwave Directions: Line 6 microwaveable muffin cups with double paper baking cups. Combine oat bran, ⅓ cup brown sugar, flour, baking powder, salt and nutmeg. Add combined milk, egg whites, oil and vanilla, mixing just until moistened. Fill muffin cups almost full. Combine oats and remaining 1 tablespoon brown sugar; sprinkle evenly over batter. Microwave at HIGH 2 minutes 30 seconds to 3 minutes or until wooden pick inserted in center comes out clean. Remove from pan; cool 5 minutes before serving. Line muffin cups with additional double paper baking cups. Repeat procedure with remaining batter.

Tips: To freeze muffins: Wrap securely in foil or place in freezer bag. Seal, label and freeze.

To reheat frozen muffins: Unwrap muffins. Microwave at HIGH about 30 seconds per muffin.

Nutrients per serving (1 muffin):

Calories	140	Sodium	90 mg
Fat	5 g	Cholesterol	0 mg

Blueberry Lover's Muffins

Low Cholesterol

Makes 12 muffins

2 cups all-purpose flour
⅓ cup sugar
4 teaspoons baking powder
1½ teaspoons cinnamon
1 teaspoon nutmeg
¼ teaspoon ginger
¼ teaspoon salt
3½ cups KELLOGG'S® 40+ BRAN-FLAKES™ cereal
2 cups skim milk
3 egg whites
3 tablespoons vegetable oil
1½ cups fresh or frozen blueberries, unthawed

1. Stir together flour, sugar, baking powder, spices and salt; set aside.

2. In large mixing bowl, combine KELLOGG'S® 40+ BRAN FLAKES™ cereal and milk. Let stand 2 minutes or until cereal is softened. Add egg whites and oil; beat well. Add dry ingredients, stirring only until combined. Gently stir in blueberries. Portion batter evenly into 12 lightly greased 2½-inch muffin-pan cups.

3. Bake in 400°F oven about 23 minutes or until light golden brown. Serve hot.

Nutrients per serving (1 muffin):

Calories	196	Sodium	299 mg
Fat	4 g	Cholesterol	0 mg

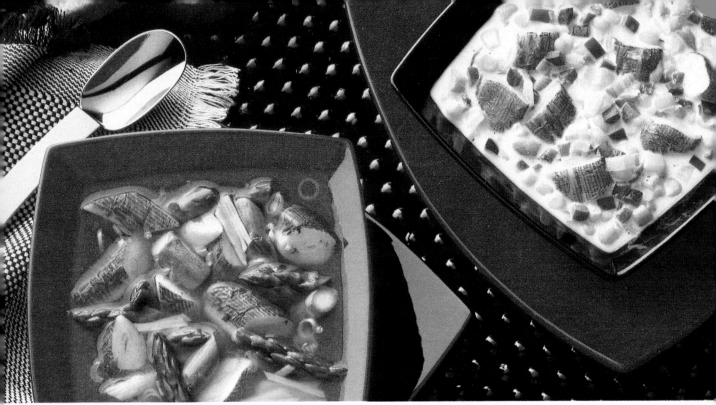

Asparagus and Surimi Seafood Soup and Seafood Corn Chowder

Seafood Corn Chowder

Low Cholesterol

Makes 6 servings.

1 tablespoon margarine
1 cup chopped onions
½ cup chopped green bell pepper
½ cup chopped red bell pepper
⅓ cup chopped celery
1 tablespoon all-purpose flour
1 can (10½ ounces) low-sodium chicken broth
2 cups skim milk
1 can (12 ounces) evaporated skim milk
8 to 12 ounces Surimi Seafood, crab flavored, chunk style
2 cups fresh or frozen whole kernel corn
½ teaspoon black pepper
½ teaspoon paprika

Melt margarine in large saucepan over medium heat. Add onions, peppers and celery. Cook, uncovered, over moderate heat for 4 to 5 minutes or until vegetables are soft. Add flour to vegetable mixture, cook and stir constantly for 2 minutes. Gradually add chicken broth and bring to a boil. Add milk, evaporated milk, Surimi Seafood, corn, black pepper and paprika. Heat, stirring occasionally, 5 minutes or until chowder is hot. Serve.

Nutrients per serving:

Calories	217	Sodium	630 mg
Fat	3 g	Cholesterol	17 mg

Favorite recipe from **National Fisheries Institute**

Asparagus and Surimi Seafood Soup

Low Cholesterol

Makes 4 servings

3 cans (10½ ounces *each*) low-sodium chicken broth (about 4 cups)
2 thin slices fresh ginger
2 cups diagonally sliced asparagus (½ inch long) (about ¾ pound)
¼ cup sliced green onions, including part of green tops
3 tablespoons rice vinegar or white wine vinegar
¼ teaspoon crushed red pepper
8 to 12 ounces Surimi Seafood, crab flavored, chunk style or leg style, cut diagonally

Bring chicken broth and ginger to a boil in a large saucepan. Add asparagus, green onions, vinegar and crushed pepper. Simmer 5 minutes or until the asparagus is crisp tender. Add Surimi Seafood and simmer 5 minutes longer or until seafood is hot. Remove and discard ginger. Serve hot.

Nutrients per serving:

Calories	136	Sodium	784 mg
Fat	3 g	Cholesterol	18 mg

Favorite recipe from **National Fisheries Institute**

Pumpkin Patch Bread

Low Sodium

Makes 2 loaves, 32 slices

1 orange
⅔ cup warm water
⅔ cup CRISCO® Shortening
2⅔ cups sugar
4 eggs
1 can (16 ounces) pumpkin
3⅓ cups all-purpose flour
2 teaspoons baking soda
2 teaspoons cinnamon
1½ teaspoons salt (optional)
½ teaspoon baking powder
⅔ cup raisins

1. Heat oven to 350°F. Grease two 9×5×3-inch loaf pans.

2. Cut orange in quarters. Remove and discard peel and white pith from sections. Place all orange sections and water in blender or food processor. Process until smooth.

3. Combine CRISCO® and sugar in large bowl. Mix with fork or spoon until blended and crumbly. Add eggs. Beat until fairly smooth. Mix in orange purée and pumpkin.

4. Combine flour, baking soda, cinnamon, salt (if used) and baking powder in separate bowl. Add to pumpkin mixture. Stir until dry ingredients are just moistened. Stir in raisins.

5. Pour evenly into pans. Bake at 350°F for 1 hour and 10 minutes. Cool 10 minutes before removing from pans. Cool completely on wire rack. Slice with serrated knife.

Nutrients per serving (1 slice):

Calories	170	Sodium	70 mg
Fat	5 g	Cholesterol	35 mg

Common Sense™ Oat Bran Bread

Low Cholesterol

Makes 1 loaf, 14 slices

1¾ cups bread flour
1 cup whole wheat flour
1½ cups KELLOGG'S® COMMON SENSE™ Oat Bran cereal, any variety
½ teaspoon salt (optional)
1 package active dry yeast
2 tablespoons firmly packed brown sugar
1 cup skim milk
¼ cup margarine
3 egg whites

1. Stir together flours. In large electric mixer bowl, combine ½ cup of the flour mixture, KELLOGG'S® COMMON SENSE™ Oat Bran cereal, salt, yeast and sugar.

2. Heat milk and margarine until very warm (120°-130°F). Gradually add to cereal mixture and beat 2 minutes on medium speed, scraping bowl occasionally. Add egg whites and 1 cup of the flour mixture. Beat 2 minutes on high speed.

3. Using dough hooks on electric mixer or by hand, stir in remaining flour mixture. Knead on low speed or by hand for 5 minutes or until dough is smooth and elastic.

4. Place dough in lightly greased bowl, turning once to coat top. Cover and let rise in warm place until double in volume. Punch down dough and let rest 10 minutes.

5. Roll dough on lightly floured surface into 14×8½-inch rectangle. Starting with short-side, roll dough lengthwise. Place seam side down in lightly greased 9×5×3-inch loaf pan. Let rise until double in volume, about 1½ hours.

6. Bake in 375°F oven about 30 minutes or until golden brown. Remove from pan and cool on wire rack.

Nutrients per serving (1 slice):

Calories	160	Sodium	110 mg
Fat	4 g	Cholesterol	0 mg

Orange Chocolate Chip Bread

Low Sodium

Makes 16 servings

1 cup skim milk
¼ cup orange juice
⅓ cup sugar
1 egg, slightly beaten
1 tablespoon grated fresh orange peel
3 cups buttermilk baking mix
½ cup HERSHEY'S® MINI CHIPS Semi-Sweet Chocolate

Combine milk, orange juice, sugar, egg and orange peel in small bowl; stir into baking mix in a medium mixing bowl. Beat until well combined, about 1 minute. Stir in MINI CHIPS. Pour into greased 9×5×3-inch loaf pan. Bake at 350° for 45 to 50 minutes or until cake tester inserted in center comes out clean. Cool 10 minutes; remove from pan. Cool completely. Slice and serve. To store leftovers, wrap in foil or plastic wrap.

Nutrients per serving (1 slice):

Calories	161	Sodium	274 mg
Fat	5 g	Cholesterol	17 mg

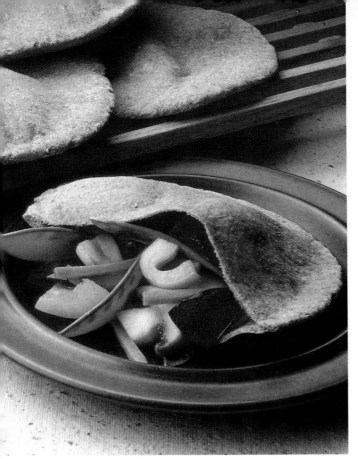

Bran Pita Bread

Bran Pita Bread

Low Cholesterol

Makes 12 servings

1 package active dry yeast
1¼ cups warm water (110°-115°F)
1½ cups KELLOGG'S® ALL-BRAN® cereal
1½ cups all-purpose flour, divided
½ teaspoon salt
¼ cup vegetable oil
1 cup whole wheat flour

1. In large bowl of electric mixer, dissolve yeast in warm water, about 5 minutes. Add KELLOGG'S® ALL-BRAN® cereal, mixing until combined. On low speed, beat in 1 cup of the all-purpose flour, the salt and oil. Beat on high speed 3 minutes, scraping sides of bowl.

2. Using dough hooks on mixer or by hand, stir in whole wheat flour. Continue kneading with mixer on low speed or by hand 5 minutes longer or until dough is smooth and elastic. Add the remaining ½ cup all-purpose flour, if needed, to make soft dough.

3. Divide dough into 12 portions. Roll each portion between floured hands into a very smooth ball. Cover with plastic wrap or a damp cloth; let rest 10 minutes.

4. On a well-floured surface, lightly roll one piece of dough at a time into 6-inch rounds, turning dough over once. Do not stretch, puncture or crease dough. Keep unrolled dough covered while rolling each dough piece. Place 2 rounds of dough at a time on ungreased baking sheet.

5. Bake in 450°F oven about 4 minutes or until dough is puffed and slightly firm. Turn with a spatula; continue baking about 2 minutes or until lightly brown; cool. Repeat with remaining dough. Cut in half and fill with a vegetable or meat filling.

Nutrients per serving (2 pita bread halves):			
Calories	160	Sodium	210 mg
Fat	5 g	Cholesterol	0 mg

Minestrone

Low Cholesterol

Makes 20 servings

2 tablespoons olive or vegetable oil
1 pound lean beef stew meat, cut into ¾-inch cubes
1 large onion, chopped
1½ cups sliced celery
2 cloves garlic, minced
10 cups water
2 tablespoons WYLER'S® Beef-Flavor Instant Bouillon
1 small head cabbage, chopped
4 medium carrots, sliced
1 can (15 ounces) chickpeas, undrained
1 can (15 ounces) kidney beans, undrained
4 medium zucchini, sliced
4 medium fresh tomatoes, peeled, seeded and chopped
1 cup chopped fresh parsley
1 teaspoon thyme leaves, crushed
1 teaspoon any salt-free herb seasoning
¼ teaspoon pepper
½ of a (1-pound) package CREAMETTE® Radiatore *or* Medium Shells, uncooked
Grated Parmesan cheese, optional

In large Dutch oven, heat oil. Add beef, onion, celery and garlic; cook until beef is no longer pink. Add water and bouillon; bring to boil. Add cabbage, carrots, chickpeas and kidney beans. Reduce heat. Cover; simmer 45 minutes. Add zucchini, tomatoes, parsley and seasonings; simmer 15 minutes longer. Prepare CREAMETTE® Radiatore or Shells as package directs; drain. Add to soup; heat through. Serve with Parmesan cheese, if desired. Refrigerate leftovers.

Nutrients per serving:			
Calories	182	Sodium	447 mg
Fat	7 g	Cholesterol	24 mg

Banana Bran Loaf

Makes 16 servings

1 cup mashed ripe bananas (about 2 large)
½ cup sugar
⅓ cup liquid vegetable oil margarine
2 egg whites
⅓ cup skim milk
1¼ cups all-purpose flour
1 cup QUAKER® Oat Bran hot cereal, uncooked
2 teaspoons baking powder
½ teaspoon baking soda

Heat oven to 350°F. Lightly spray 8×4-inch or 9×5-inch loaf pan with vegetable oil cooking spray or oil lightly. Combine bananas, sugar, margarine, egg whites and milk; mix well. Add combined flour, oat bran, baking powder and baking soda, mixing just until moistened. Pour into prepared pan. Bake 55 to 60 minutes or until wooden pick inserted in center comes out clean. Cool 10 minutes in pan; remove to wire rack. Cool completely.

Tips: To freeze bread slices: Layer waxed paper between each slice of bread. Wrap securely in foil or place in freezer bag. Seal, label and freeze.

To reheat bread slices: Unwrap frozen bread slices; wrap in paper towel. Microwave at HIGH about 30 seconds for each slice, or until warm.

Nutrients per serving (1 slice):			
Calories	130	Sodium	110 mg
Fat	4 g	Cholesterol	0 mg

Banana Bran Loaf

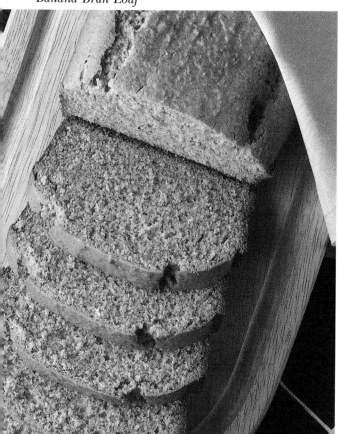

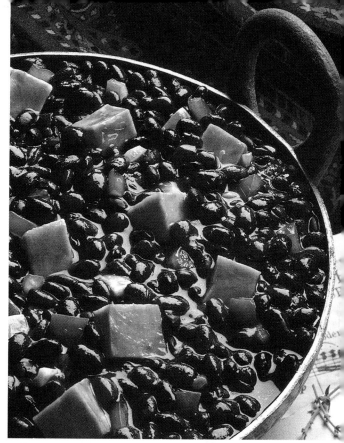

Cuban Black Bean & Ham Soup

Cuban Black Bean & Ham Soup

Makes 4 servings

1 cup uncooked black beans, soaked overnight and drained
1 slice (2 ounces) ARMOUR® Lower Salt Ham
½ cup chopped green bell pepper
1 medium onion, finely chopped
2 teaspoons MRS. DASH® original blend
1 teaspoon garlic powder
1 teaspoon ground cumin
¼ teaspoon black pepper
1½ cups (6 ounces) ARMOUR® Lower Salt Ham cut into ¾-inch cubes

Combine beans, ham slice, green pepper, onion and seasonings in medium saucepan; add enough water to just cover beans. Bring to boil; reduce heat, cover and simmer about 1½ to 2 hours, or until beans are tender and most of liquid is absorbed. Add ham cubes. Cook 10 minutes, or until ham is heated through. Remove ham slice before serving. Serve over rice, if desired.

Nutrients per serving:			
Calories	244	Sodium	489 mg
Fat	4 g	Cholesterol	28 mg

Vegetable and Ham Soup

Makes 6 to 8 servings

2 tablespoons unsalted margarine or butter
1 medium onion, coarsely chopped
1 large potato, peeled and diced
1 package (16 ounces) frozen mixed vegetables
2½ cups (10 ounces) ARMOUR® Lower Salt Ham, cut into ½-inch cubes
2½ tablespoons no salt added chicken flavor instant bouillon
2 teaspoons MRS. DASH®, original blend
Pepper to taste

Melt margarine in Dutch oven over medium heat. Add onion; sauté until tender. Add remaining ingredients and 5 cups water. Bring to boil over medium-high heat. Reduce heat to simmer. Cook, uncovered, for 30 minutes, or until potato is tender. Garnish with carrot curls and fresh chives, if desired.

Microwave Directions: Place margarine and onion in 10-inch microwave-safe tube pan. Cover with vented plastic wrap; cook on High power about 2 to 3 minutes, or until onion is tender. Add remaining ingredients and 5 cups water. Cover with vented plastic wrap. Cook on High power for 10 minutes, or until boiling. Reduce power to Medium-High (70%); continue cooking for 30 minutes, or until potato is tender. Garnish as above.

Nutrients per serving:			
Calories	157	Sodium	334 mg
Fat	6 g	Cholesterol	18 mg

Vegetable and Ham Soup

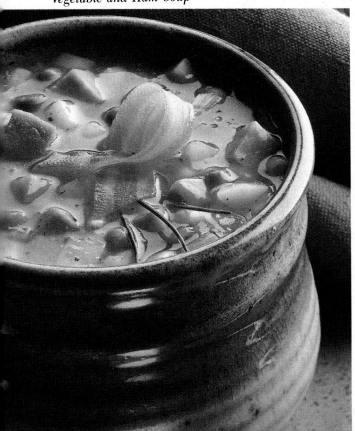

Apple Streusel Coffee Cake

Makes 9 servings

Cake
¼ cup CRISCO® Shortening
½ cup sugar
2 egg whites
1 teaspoon vanilla
¾ cup dry oat bran high fiber hot cereal
1 cup chunky applesauce
1¼ cups all-purpose flour
1½ teaspoons cinnamon
1 teaspoon baking powder
¾ teaspoon baking soda
¼ teaspoon salt (optional)
¼ teaspoon nutmeg

Filling and Topping
1 cup chunky applesauce, divided
¼ cup sugar
¼ teaspoon cinnamon

1. Heat oven to 375°F. Grease 8-inch square pan.

2. For cake: Cream CRISCO® and sugar in medium bowl with fork until blended and crumbly. Add egg whites and vanilla. Beat until fairly smooth. Stir in oat bran and applesauce. Let stand 5 minutes.

3. Combine flour, cinnamon, baking powder, baking soda, salt (if used) and nutmeg in separate bowl. Stir into oat bran mixture. Spread half of batter in pan.

4. For filling and topping: Spread ¾ cup applesauce over batter. Combine sugar and cinnamon. Sprinkle half over applesauce. Add remaining batter, gently spreading evenly. Top with remaining ¼ cup applesauce. Spread thinly and evenly. Sprinkle with remaining sugar and cinnamon mixture.

5. Bake at 375°F for 30 to 35 minutes or until top is golden brown and center springs back when touched lightly. Cut in squares. Serve warm.

Nutrients per serving:			
Calories	250	Sodium	130 mg
Fat	6 g	Cholesterol	0 mg

Baking Powder Biscuits

Makes 12 biscuits

1½ cups all-purpose flour
¼ cup sugar
2½ teaspoons baking powder
½ teaspoon salt (optional)
2 tablespoons plus 2 teaspoons CRISCO® Shortening
½ cup skim milk
Skim milk for brushing tops

1. Heat oven to 450°F.

2. Combine flour, sugar, baking powder and salt (if used) in medium bowl. Cut in CRISCO® with pastry blender (or 2 knives) to form coarse crumbs.

3. Add milk. Stir until dry ingredients are just moistened. Place on floured surface. Pat or roll into circle slightly more than ½-inch thick°.

4. With 2-inch round biscuit cutter, cut 8 or 9 biscuits. Press dough scraps into ball. Flatten again. Cut remaining 3 or 4 biscuits. Place on ungreased baking sheet. Brush tops with milk.

5. Bake at 450°F for 6 to 8 minutes or until tops begin to brown. Serve warm.

°*Hint: Cover dough with waxed paper. Press and flatten with 8- or 9-inch round cake pan until dough is desired thickness.*

Nutrients per serving (1 biscuit):

Calories	100	Sodium	115 mg
Fat	3 g	Cholesterol	0 mg

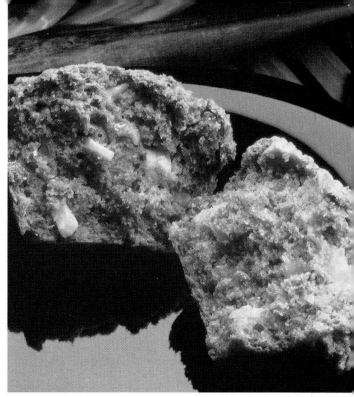

Papaya Muffins

Chicken Lemon Soup Oriental

Quick & Easy

Makes 6 servings

1 can (16 ounces) California cling peach halves in juice or extra light syrup
8 cups water
2 chicken flavored bouillon cubes
2 cloves garlic, minced
1 pound skinless, boneless chicken breasts
¼ cup long grain white rice
2 cups fresh mushroom caps, cut in half
⅓ cup *each* sliced green onions and chopped cilantro
¼ cup lemon juice
1 tablespoon grated fresh ginger
¼ teaspoon red pepper flakes (optional)

Drain peaches, reserving all liquid. Dice peaches and set aside. Combine peach liquid with water, bouillon cubes and garlic. Bring to a boil; stir in chicken and rice. Simmer 15 minutes, or until chicken is cooked through. Remove chicken and chop into bite-size pieces. Stir chicken, reserved diced peaches and remaining ingredients into soup. Simmer 5 minutes.

Nutrients per serving:

Calories	160	Sodium	318 mg
Fat	1 g	Cholesterol	44 mg

Favorite recipe from **California Cling Peach Advisory Board**

Papaya Muffins

Low Sodium

Makes 12 Muffins

1½ cups whole wheat flour
1 tablespoon baking powder
½ teaspoon salt
1½ cups KELLOGG'S® ALL-BRAN® cereal
1¼ cups skim milk
¼ cup honey
¼ cup vegetable oil
1 tablespoon dark molasses
1 egg
¾ cup chopped fresh papaya
2 teaspoons finely chopped crystallized ginger

1. Stir together flour, baking powder and salt. Set aside.

2. Measure KELLOGG'S® ALL-BRAN® cereal and milk into large mixing bowl. Let stand 2 minutes or until cereal is softened. Add honey, oil, molasses and egg. Beat well. Stir in papaya and ginger.

3. Add flour mixture, stirring only until combined. Portion batter evenly into 12 greased 2½-inch muffin-pan cups.

4. Bake at 400°F about 25 minutes or until muffins are golden brown. Serve warm.

Nutrients per serving (1 muffin):

Calories	160	Sodium	314 mg
Fat	6 g	Cholesterol	19 mg

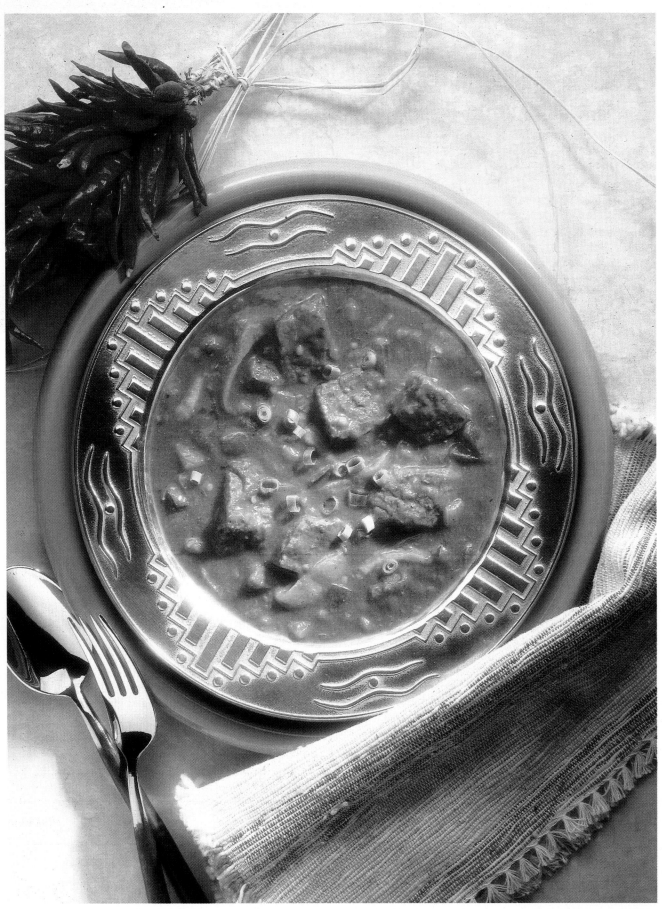

Southwestern Beef Stew

Main Dishes

Southwestern Beef Stew

Makes 4 servings

1¼ pounds well-trimmed beef tip roast, cut into
    1-inch pieces
1 tablespoon vegetable oil
½ cup coarsely chopped onion
1 large clove garlic, minced
1½ teaspoons dried oregano leaves
1 teaspoon ground cumin
½ teaspoon *each* crushed red pepper and salt
4 medium tomatoes, chopped and divided (about
    4 cups)
½ cup water
1 can (4 ounces) whole green chilies
1 tablespoon cornstarch
¼ cup sliced green onion tops

Heat oil in Dutch oven over medium-high heat. Add
beef pieces, onion and garlic; cook and stir until beef
is browned. Pour off drippings. Combine oregano,
cumin, red pepper and salt; sprinkle over beef. Add 3
cups of the tomatoes and the water, stirring to
combine. Reduce heat; cover tightly and simmer 1
hour and 55 minutes or until beef is tender, stirring
occasionally. Drain green chilies; reserve liquid. Cut
chilies into ½-inch pieces; add to beef mixture.
Combine cornstarch and reserved liquid; gradually
stir into stew and cook, uncovered, until thickened.
Stir in remaining tomatoes; garnish with green onion
tops.

Nutrients per serving:			
Calories	250	Sodium	546 mg
Fat	8 g	Cholesterol	85 mg

Favorite recipe from **National Livestock and Meat Board**

Oriental Almond Stir-Fry

Quick & Easy

Makes 4 servings

2 tablespoons dry sherry
1 tablespoon soy sauce
½ teaspoon sugar
¼ teaspoon ground ginger
1 clove garlic, minced
¾ pound shrimp, peeled and deveined
1 tablespoon vegetable oil, divided
2 cups diagonally sliced celery, ¼-inch
2 cups fresh mushrooms, sliced
1 tablespoon cornstarch
6 tablespoons water
1 package (10 ounces) frozen peas (about 2 cups)
1½ cups bean sprouts
¼ cup BLUE DIAMOND® Blanched Whole
    Almonds

Make marinade by combining first five ingredients in
a medium bowl. Add shrimp and let stand at least 10
minutes, stirring occasionally. Using heavy non-stick
skillet or wok, heat 1½ teaspoons oil over medium-
high heat. Add celery and stir-fry 1 minute. Remove
from pan and set aside. Heat remaining 1½ teaspoons
oil. With slotted spoon, remove shrimp from marinade
and stir-fry 2 to 3 minutes, or until shrimp turn pink.
Add mushrooms and stir-fry 2 to 3 minutes, adding 1
tablespoon water if necessary to prevent sticking. Stir
cornstarch and 6 tablespoons water into marinade;
add to skillet and cook about 30 seconds, until
thickened. Add celery and remaining ingredients and
stir-fry 3 to 4 minutes, until bean sprouts are soft, but
still crisp. Serve over hot brown rice, if desired.

Nutrients per serving:			
Calories	275	Sodium	585 mg
Fat	10 g	Cholesterol	165 mg

Confetti Scallops & Noodles

Makes 8 servings

½ of a (1-pound) package CREAMETTE® Egg
   Noodles, uncooked
1 cup water
2 teaspoons WYLER'S® Chicken-Flavor Instant
   Bouillon
½ cup dry white wine
2 tablespoons lemon juice
2 cloves garlic, minced
1 teaspoon dill weed
½ teaspoon lemon pepper seasoning
1 pound bay scallops
2 cups shredded cabbage
1 cup sliced carrots
½ cup sliced green onions
3 cups torn fresh spinach leaves

Prepare CREAMETTE® Egg Noodles as package
directs; drain. In large non-stick skillet, bring water
and bouillon to boil. Reduce heat; add remaining
ingredients except spinach and noodles. Cover;
simmer 10 minutes. Add spinach; cook and stir 5
minutes longer. Toss with hot cooked noodles. Serve
immediately. Refrigerate leftovers.

*Note: To reduce sodium, substitute low-sodium
bouillon.*

Nutrients per serving:			
Calories	207	Sodium	293 mg
Fat	2 g	Cholesterol	30 mg

Confetti Scallops & Noodles

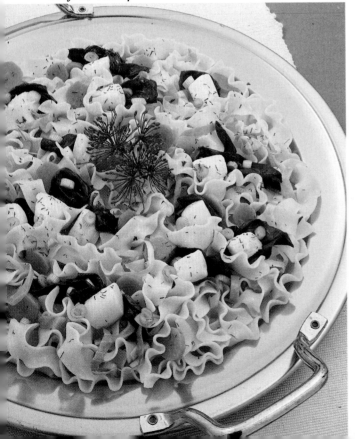

Lasagna

Makes 12 servings

1 cup chopped onions
3 cloves garlic, minced
2 tablespoons PURITAN® Oil
1 pound extra-lean ground beef
2 cans (14½ ounces *each*) no-salt-added stewed
   tomatoes
1 can (6 ounces) no-salt-added tomato paste
2 teaspoons dried basil leaves
1 teaspoon dried oregano leaves
½ teaspoon sugar
¼ teaspoon pepper
2 cups low-fat cottage cheese
½ cup grated Parmesan cheese, divided
¼ cup chopped parsley
8 ounces wide lasagna noodles
1 cup shredded low moisture part-skim
   mozzarella cheese, divided

1. Sauté onions and garlic in PURITAN® Oil in large
skillet on medium heat until soft. Push to one side of
skillet. Add ground beef. Cook, stirring well, to
crumble beef. Drain, if necessary. Add tomatoes.
Break into smaller pieces. Add tomato paste, basil,
oregano, sugar and pepper. Simmer 30 minutes.

2. Combine cottage cheese, ¼ cup Parmesan cheese
and parsley. Set aside.

3. Cook lasagna noodles 7 minutes in unsalted boiling
water. Drain well.

4. Heat oven to 350°F.

5. Place thin layer of meat sauce in 13×9×2-inch
pan. Add in layers half the noodles, half the cottage
cheese mixture, 2 tablespoons Parmesan cheese, ⅓
cup mozzarella, and thin layer of sauce. Repeat
noodle and cheese layers. Top with remaining sauce
and remaining ⅓ cup mozzarella.

6. Bake at 350°F for 45 minutes. Let stand 15 minutes
before serving. Cut in rectangles about 3×4 inches.

Nutrients per serving:			
Calories	270	Sodium	300 mg
Fat	10 g	Cholesterol	55 mg

Brunch Potato Cassoulet

Low Cholesterol

Makes 4 to 6 servings

2 tablespoons unsalted margarine or butter
2 cups (8 ounces) ARMOUR® Lower Salt Ham,
    cut into ½-inch cubes
2 cups frozen natural potato wedges
1 cup sliced mushrooms
½ cup chopped red onion
½ cup chopped green bell pepper
1 cup frozen speckled butter beans, cooked
    according to package directions omitting salt
    and drained
    Lower salt cheese (optional)

Preheat oven to 350°F. Melt margarine in large skillet over medium heat. Add ham, potatoes, mushrooms, onion and green bell pepper; cook over medium heat about 5 to 6 minutes, or until onion is soft. Stir in cooked beans. Transfer to medium earthenware pot or ovenproof Dutch oven. Bake, covered, about 10 to 12 minutes, or until heated through. If desired, sprinkle with lower salt cheese and broil 4 to 6 inches from heat source about 2 to 3 minutes, or until cheese is melted and slightly browned.

Nutrients per serving:

Calories	161	Sodium	391 mg
Fat	7 g	Cholesterol	19 mg

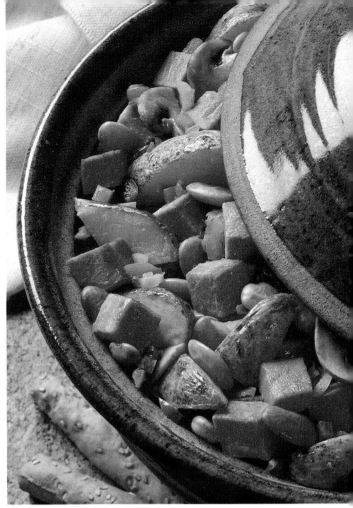

Brunch Potato Cassoulet

Oven Campout Fish with BBQ Sauce

Quick & Easy

Makes 4 servings

¼ cup minced onion
1 clove garlic, minced
1 teaspoon margarine
1 can (8 ounces) DOLE® Pineapple Tidbits
½ cup bottled barbecue sauce
1 tablespoon brown sugar *or* honey
4 cod or red snapper fillets (1 pound)
1 tablespoon vegetable oil
    Juice from 1 lemon

In skillet, sauté onion and garlic in margarine until soft. Add undrained pineapple with juice, barbecue sauce and brown sugar. Cook over medium heat, stirring, until thickened and slightly reduced. Brush fish with oil. Sprinkle with lemon juice. Broil 4 to 6 inches from heat 5 minutes. Turn fish and continue cooking 5 to 7 minutes longer until fish is done. Serve fish with barbecue sauce.

Nutrients per serving:

Calories	238	Sodium	356 mg
Fat	6 g	Cholesterol	63 mg

Tacos de Queso

Low Cholesterol

Makes 6 servings

1 can (15 ounces) refried beans
1½ cups LIGHT N'LIVELY® Cottage Cheese
1 cup (4 ounces) shredded KRAFT® Light
    Naturals Reduced Fat Mild Cheddar Cheese
1 can (4 ounces) green chilies, drained
½ teaspoon chili powder
12 taco shells
    Shredded lettuce
    Chopped tomatoes

Preheat oven to 350°F. Heat beans according to label directions. Combine cheeses, chilies and chili powder; mix well. Fill each taco shell with approximately 3 tablespoons beans and ¼ cup cheese mixture. Place tacos in 13×9-inch baking dish. Bake 10 to 15 minutes or until thoroughly heated. Top with lettuce and tomatoes.

Nutrients per serving:

Calories	250	Sodium	610 mg
Fat	10 g	Cholesterol	20 mg

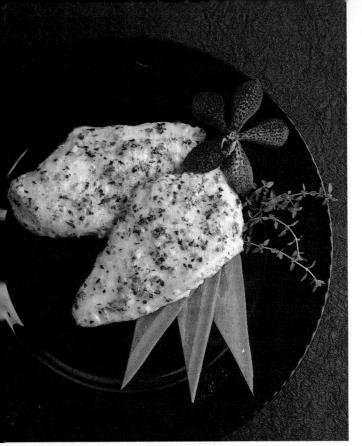

Herb-Marinated Chicken Breasts

Dieter's Fish and Spinach

Quick & Easy

Makes 2 servings

2 (4 ounces *each*) frozen sole fillets, thawed
1 tablespoon REALEMON® Lemon Juice from
    Concentrate
Salt and pepper
1 package (10 ounces) frozen chopped spinach,
    cooked and well drained
¼ cup BORDEN® Lite-line® skim milk
2 slices BORDEN® Lite-line® Process Cheese
    Product (any flavor), cut into small pieces°
Paprika

Preheat oven to 400°. Brush fillets with ReaLemon®
lemon juice; sprinkle lightly with salt and pepper.
Spread spinach over bottom of 8-inch shallow baking
dish. Pour milk over spinach; top with Lite-line®
pieces, then fillets. Cover; bake 20 minutes or until
fish flakes with fork. Sprinkle with paprika.
Refrigerate leftovers.

°"½ the calories" 8% milkfat version

Nutrients per serving:

Calories	182	Sodium	716 mg
Fat	4 g	Cholesterol	65 mg

Herb-Marinated Chicken Breasts

Quick & Easy

Makes 6 servings

¾ cup MIRACLE WHIP® Salad dressing
¼ cup dry white wine
2 garlic cloves, minced
2 tablespoons finely chopped green onion
2 teaspoons dried basil leaves, crushed
1 teaspoon dried thyme leaves, crushed
3 whole chicken breasts, split, boned, skinned

Stir together dressing, wine, garlic, onion and
seasonings. Pour dressing mixture over chicken.
Cover; marinate in refrigerator several hours or
overnight. Drain, reserving dressing mixture. Place
chicken on greased rack of broiler pan. Broil 4 to 6
minutes on each side or until tender, brushing
frequently with dressing mixture.

*Variations: For outdoor grilling: Place chicken on
greased grill over low coals (coals will be ash gray).
Grill, uncovered, 4 to 6 minutes on each side or until
tender, brushing frequently with dressing mixture.*

Nutrients per serving:

Calories	170	Sodium	110 mg
Fat	7 g	Cholesterol	55 mg

Spaghetti With Pesto Sauce

Low Sodium

Makes 10 servings

1 package (1-pound) CREAMETTE® Spaghetti,
    uncooked
2 cups tightly packed fresh basil leaves
2 tablespoons pine nuts
¼ cup olive oil
⅓ cup freshly grated Parmesan cheese
2 cloves garlic, minced

Prepare CREAMETTE® Spaghetti as package directs;
drain. In blender or food processor, combine
remaining ingredients; process until smooth. Toss
pesto sauce with hot cooked spaghetti. Serve
immediately. Refrigerate leftovers.

Nutrients per serving:

Calories	260	Sodium	63 mg
Fat	8 g	Cholesterol	3 mg

Southwest Vegetable Chili

Low Cholesterol

Makes 4 servings

1 cup coarsely chopped onions
1 medium green bell pepper, cut into ½-inch
    pieces
2 cloves garlic, minced
½ cup water
2 beef bouillon cubes
1 tablespoon chili powder
½ teaspoon cumin
¼ cup HEINZ® Wine Vinegar
1 can (15½ ounces) kidney beans
1 can (14½ ounces) tomatoes, cut into bite-size
    pieces
1 can (11 ounces) whole kernel corn, drained
    Hot cooked rice

In 3-quart saucepan, combine first 7 ingredients; simmer, covered, 5 minutes or until vegetables are tender. Stir in vinegar, beans, tomatoes and corn. Bring mixture to a boil; simmer, uncovered, 30 minutes, stirring occasionally. To serve, spoon vegetable chili into individual bowls and top with rice.

Nutrients per serving:

Calories	232	Sodium	1155 mg
Fat	0 g	Cholesterol	0 mg

Orange Roughy with Cucumber Relish

Low Sodium

Makes 4 servings

1 can (11 ounces) mandarin oranges, drained
1 small cucumber, peeled, seeded, finely chopped
⅓ cup HEINZ® Distilled White Vinegar
1 green onion, minced
1 tablespoon snipped fresh dill *or* 1 teaspoon
    dried dill weed
    Nonstick cooking spray
4 orange roughy fillets (about 5 ounces *each*)
    Dill sprigs

Reserve 8 orange sections for garnish; coarsely chop remaining sections and combine with cucumber, vinegar, onion and dill. Spray broiler pan with cooking spray; place fish on pan. Spoon 1 tablespoon liquid from cucumber mixture over each fillet. Broil, 3 to 4 inches from heat source, 8 to 10 minutes or until fish is cooked. To serve, spoon cucumber relish on top of fish. Garnish with reserved orange sections and dill sprigs.

Nutrients per serving:

Calories	229	Sodium	95 mg
Fat	10 g	Cholesterol	28 mg

Orange Roughy with Cucumber Relish

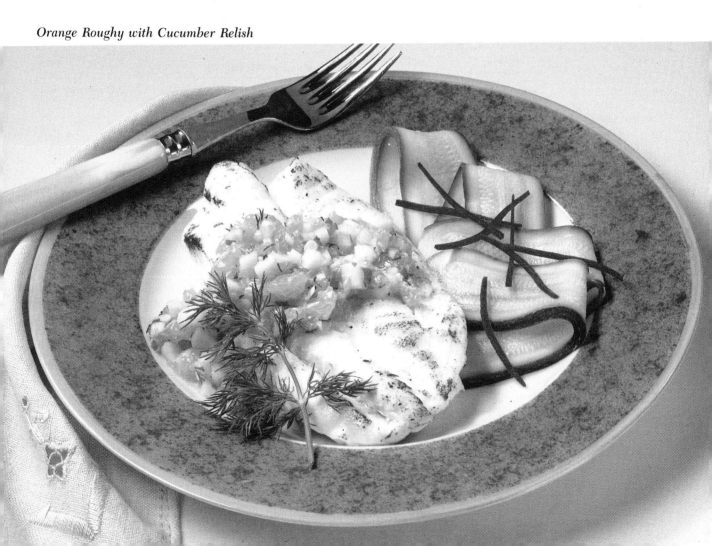

Tuna Veronique

Quick & Easy

Makes 4 servings

2 leeks or green onions
1 tablespoon vegetable oil
½ cup thin carrot strips
1 stalk celery, cut diagonally into slices
1¾ cups or 1 can (14½ ounces) chicken broth
2 tablespoons cornstarch
⅓ cup dry white wine
1¼ cups seedless red and green grapes, cut into halves
1 can (12½ ounces) STARKIST® Tuna, drained and broken into chunks
1 tablespoon chopped chives
¼ teaspoon white or black pepper
4 to 5 slices bread, toasted and cut into quarters or 8 to 10 slices toasted French bread

If using leeks, wash thoroughly between leaves. Cut off white portion; trim and slice ¼-inch thick. Discard green portion. For green onions, trim and slice ¼-inch thick. In a large nonstick skillet sauté leeks, carrots and celery in oil for 3 minutes. In a small bowl stir together chicken broth and cornstarch until smooth; stir into vegetables. Cook and stir until mixture thickens and bubbles. Stir in wine; simmer for 2 minutes. Stir in grapes, tuna, chives and pepper. Cook for 2 minutes more to heat through. To serve, ladle sauce over toast points.

Nutrients per serving:			
Calories	273	Sodium	886 mg
Fat	5 g	Cholesterol	39 mg

Tuna Veronique

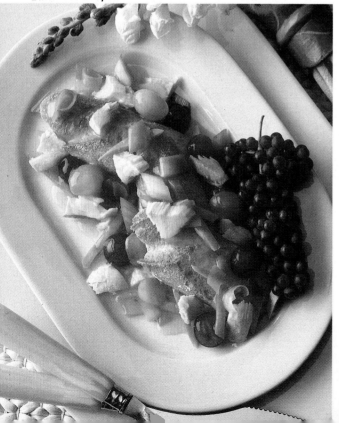

Sweet Sour Chicken Sauté

Low Sodium

Makes 4 servings

1 can (8 ounces) pineapple chunks
1 tablespoon cornstarch
⅓ cup HEINZ® Apple Cider Vinegar
¼ cup firmly packed brown sugar
⅛ teaspoon pepper
1 small red bell pepper, cut into thin strips
1 small green bell pepper, cut into thin strips
1 medium onion, thinly sliced
1 pound skinless boneless chicken breasts, cut into ½-inch strips

Drain pineapple; reserve juice. Combine juice with cornstarch and next 3 ingredients; set aside. Spray large skillet with cooking spray. Sauté peppers and onion until tender-crisp; remove. Spray skillet again; sauté chicken 2 to 3 minutes or until chicken changes color. Stir in reserved vinegar mixture; cook 2 to 3 minutes or until chicken is cooked and sauce is thickened. Add vegetables and pineapple; heat, stirring occasionally. Serve with rice if desired.

Nutrients per serving:			
Calories	225	Sodium	83 mg
Fat	2 g	Cholesterol	68 mg

Two-Cheese Enchiladas

Low Cholesterol

Makes 4 servings

1 cup salsa, divided
1½ cups LIGHT N' LIVELY® Cottage Cheese
1 cup shredded KRAFT® Light Naturals Reduced Fat Cheddar Cheese, divided
¼ cup green onion slices
¼ teaspoon dried oregano leaves, crushed
8 (6-inch) flour tortillas, warmed

Preheat oven to 375°. Spread ¼ cup salsa in 12×8-inch baking dish. Combine cottage cheese, ½ cup cheddar cheese, onions and oregano. Fill each tortilla with ¼ cup cheese mixture in center of each tortilla; roll up. Place, seam side down, over salsa. Top with remaining ½ cup cheddar cheese and ¾ cup salsa. Cover. Bake 20 to 25 minutes or until thoroughly heated.

Nutrients per serving:			
Calories	260	Sodium	850 mg
Fat	8 g	Cholesterol	30 mg

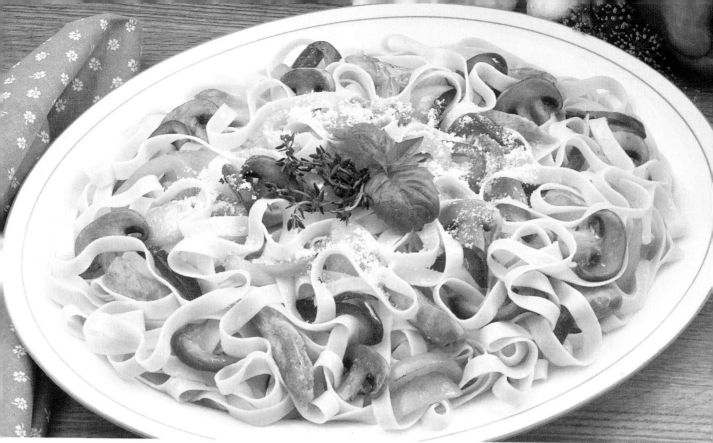

Pepper-Chicken Fettuccini Toss

Pepper-Chicken Fettuccini Toss

Low Sodium

Makes 12 servings

1 package (1 pound) CREAMETTE® Fettuccini, uncooked
¼ cup olive or vegetable oil
3 whole boneless skinless chicken breasts, cut into strips (about 18 ounces)
2 large red bell peppers, cut into strips
2 large yellow bell peppers, cut into strips
1 medium green bell pepper, cut into strips
1 medium onion, cut into chunks
2 cups sliced fresh mushrooms
1 teaspoon any salt-free herb seasoning
2 tablespoons grated Parmesan cheese

Prepare CREAMETTE® Fettuccini as package directs; drain. In large skillet, heat oil; add chicken, peppers, onion, mushrooms and seasoning. Cook and stir over medium heat until chicken is cooked through, 8 to 10 minutes. Add hot cooked fettuccini and Parmesan cheese; toss to coat. Serve immediately. Refrigerate leftovers.

Nutrients per serving:			
Calories	264	Sodium	33 mg
Fat	7 g	Cholesterol	36 mg

Stuffed Chicken Breasts

Makes 4 servings

4 (4-ounce) skinless boneless chicken breast halves, pounded flat
Pepper
8 slices BORDEN® Lite-line® Process Cheese Product, any flavor°
1 package (9 ounces) frozen French-style green beans, thawed and drained
2 tablespoons chopped pimento
1 can (8 ounces) tomato sauce
½ teaspoon oregano leaves

Preheat oven to 350°. Season chicken with pepper. Top each chicken piece with 2 Lite-line slices. Combine beans and pimento; place about ½ cup on each chicken piece. Bring ends of chicken together; secure with wooden picks. Place in 8-inch square baking dish. Combine tomato sauce and oregano; pour over chicken. Cover; bake 30 minutes. Uncover and bake 10 minutes longer. To serve, remove picks and spoon sauce over chicken. Refrigerate leftovers.

°"½ the calories" 8% milkfat version

Nutrients per serving:			
Calories	249	Sodium	1068 mg
Fat	6 g	Cholesterol	88 mg

Poached Turkey Tenderloins with Tarragon Sauce

Makes 4 servings

1 to 1½ pounds turkey tenderloins
¾ cup white wine
½ cup chopped celery
¼ cup sliced green onions
3 tablespoons chopped fresh tarragon *or*
    1 teaspoon dry, crushed tarragon
½ teaspoon salt
¼ teaspoon white pepper
  Water
  Tarragon Sauce (recipe follows)
  Steamed spinach

In a large skillet, arrange tenderloins in a single layer. Add wine, celery, onions, spices and enough water to cover tenderloins. Cover skillet and poach over low heat about 40 minutes or until no longer pink in center. Remove tenderloins, reserving poaching liquid for Tarragon Sauce°.

Microwave Directions: In 1-quart microwave-safe dish, combine celery, onions, spices and wine. Arrange tenderloins in a circle, overlapping thin ends. Cover with vented plastic wrap. Microwave at High (100% power) 5 to 6 minutes per pound or until tenderloins are no longer pink in center. Turn tenderloins over halfway through cooking time.

Tarragon Sauce

  Reserved poaching liquid
3 tablespoons cold water
2 tablespoons cornstarch
2 tablespoons chopped fresh tarragon *or*
    ½ teaspoon dry crushed tarragon
½ cup plain low-fat yogurt
1 tablespoon chopped parsley
1 tablespoon lemon juice

In a saucepan over high heat, bring reserved poaching liquid to boil for 5 to 10 minutes to reduce liquid; strain. Measure 2 cups liquid and return to saucepan. Bring to boil. Combine cold water and cornstarch. Stir into boiling liquid. Reduce heat and add tarragon. Over low heat, cook sauce until slightly thickened. Stir in yogurt, parsley and lemon juice. Slice tenderloins into ½-inch medallions. To serve, arrange medallions on steamed spinach. Drizzle with sauce. Garnish with strips of lemon peel, if desired.

°Note: Recipe may be prepared to this point, cooled, covered and refrigerated for up to two days.

Nutrients per serving:			
Calories	203	Sodium	405 mg
Fat	3 g	Cholesterol	90 mg

Favorite recipe from **National Turkey Federation**

Fast Beef Roast with Mushroom Sauce

Makes 6 to 8 servings

1 boneless beef rib eye roast (about 2 pounds)
2 tablespoons vegetable oil
4 cups water
1 can (10¾ ounces) condensed beef broth
1 cup dry red wine
2 cloves garlic, minced
1 teaspoon dried marjoram leaves
4 black peppercorns
3 whole cloves
  Mushroom Sauce (recipe follows)

Tie roast with heavy string at 2-inch intervals. Heat oil in Dutch oven over medium-high heat. Cook roast until evenly browned. Pour off drippings. Add water, broth, wine, garlic, marjoram, peppercorns and cloves; bring to boil. Reduce heat to medium-low; cover, simmer 15 minutes per pound. Check temperature with instant-read thermometer; temperature should be 130°F for rare. *Do not overcook.* Remove roast to serving platter; reserve cooking liquid. Cover roast tightly with plastic wrap or foil; allow to stand 10 minutes before carving (temperature will continue to rise about 10°F to 140°F for rare). Prepare Mushroom Sauce. Remove strings from roast. Carve into thin slices and top with Mushroom Sauce. Serve with assorted vegetables, if desired.

Note: A boneless beef rib eye roast will yield three to four 3-ounce cooked servings per pound.

Mushroom Sauce

1 tablespoon butter
1 cup sliced fresh mushrooms
1 cup beef cooking liquid, strained
1½ teaspoons cornstarch
¼ teaspoon salt
2 dashes pepper
1 tablespoon thinly sliced green onion tops

Melt butter in medium saucepan over medium-high heat. Add mushrooms; cook and stir 5 minutes. Remove and reserve. Add cooking liquid, cornstarch, salt and pepper to pan. Bring to a boil; cook and stir until thickened, 1 to 2 minutes. Remove from heat. Stir in reserved mushrooms and the green onion.

Nutrients per serving (includes 3 tablespoons sauce):			
Calories	188	Sodium	327 mg
Fat	8 g	Cholesterol	59 mg

Favorite recipe from **National Livestock and Meat Board**

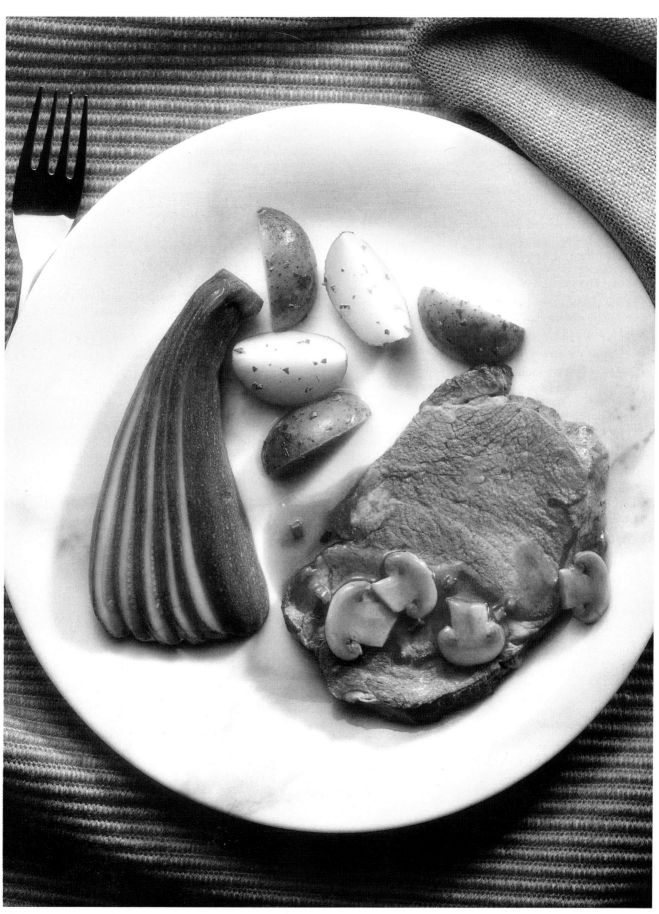

Fast Beef Roast with Mushroom Sauce

Chicken Pasta

Low Cholesterol

Makes 6 servings

2 skinless boneless chicken breasts, about
   6 ounces *each*
1 tablespoon Chef Paul Prudhomme's MEAT
   MAGIC®, in all
6 ounces pasta (fettucini or angel hair work well,
   but use your favorite)
1 cup chopped onions
½ cup chopped celery
½ cup chopped green bell pepper
2 cups defatted chicken stock, in all
2 tablespoons flour
3 cups thinly sliced fresh mushrooms
1 teaspoon minced garlic
½ cup chopped green onions

Cut the chicken into thin strips, place in a small bowl
and combine thoroughly with 2 teaspoons of the
MEAT MAGIC®.

Cook pasta according to package directions.

Place skillet over high heat and add the onions, celery,
bell pepper and the remaining teaspoon of MEAT
MAGIC®. Cook over high heat, shaking pan and
stirring occasionally (don't scrape!) for 5 minutes. Add
½ cup chicken stock, scrape up the browned coating
on the bottom of the pan and cook another 4 minutes.
Stir in the chicken mixture and cook 4 minutes. Add
the flour and stir well, cooking another 2 minutes.
Now add the mushrooms and garlic, folding in
carefully so mushrooms don't break. Add ½ cup
chicken stock and scrape up the pan bottom. Cook 4
minutes and add another ½ cup stock, stirring and
scraping. Continue cooking another 5 minutes, then
add the green onions and the remaining ½ cup stock.
Stir and scrape well. Cook 5 more minutes and
remove from heat.

To serve: Place a scant cup of pasta on each plate and
top with ½ cup of the chicken mixture.

Nutrients per serving:			
Calories	219	Sodium	593 mg
Fat	3 g	Cholesterol	49 mg

Pork Loin Roulade

Quick & Easy

Makes 4 servings

4 boneless center pork loin slices, about one
   pound
½ red bell pepper, cut into strips
½ green bell pepper, cut into strips
1 tablespoon vegetable oil
⅔ cup orange juice
⅔ cup bottled barbecue sauce
1 tablespoon prepared Dijon-style mustard

Place cutlets between 2 pieces of plastic wrap. Pound
with a mallet to about ¼-inch thickness.

Place several red and green pepper strips crosswise on
each pork portion; roll up jelly-roll style. Secure rolls
with wooden toothpicks.

In a large heavy skillet, brown the pork rolls in hot oil.
Drain fat from pan. Combine remaining ingredients
and add to skillet. Bring mixture to boiling; reduce
heat. Cover and simmer 10 to 12 minutes or until
pork is tender. Remove toothpicks and serve.

Nutrients per serving:			
Calories	255	Sodium	530 mg
Fat	10 g	Cholesterol	72 mg

Favorite recipe from **National Pork Producers Council**

Pork Loin Roulade

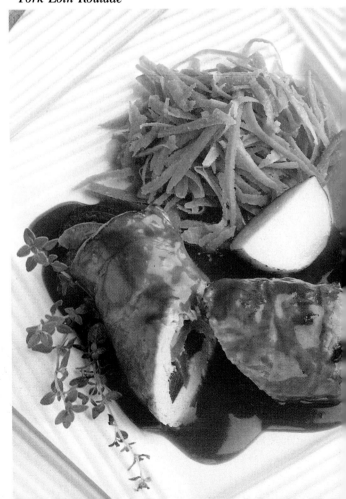

Pasta Primavera

Quick & Easy

Makes 6 servings

1 cup WISH-BONE® Lite Italian Dressing
½ cup finely chopped green onions
   Assorted fresh vegetables°
4 medium tomatoes, chopped
¼ cup dry white wine (optional)
2 tablespoons finely chopped fresh basil leaves
   (optional)
1 teaspoon LAWRY'S® Seasoned Salt
¼ teaspoon LAWRY'S® Seasoned Pepper
1 pound fettuccini noodles, cooked and drained

In 3-quart microwave-safe casserole, microwave Italian dressing, green onions and carrots (if used), covered, at High (full power) 4 minutes, stirring once. Add remaining assorted fresh vegetables and microwave, covered, at High 3½ minutes. Stir in tomatoes and microwave, covered, at High 4 minutes or until vegetables are crisp-tender. Stir in wine, basil, seasoned salt and seasoned pepper and microwave, uncovered, at High 2 minutes, stirring once. Toss with hot fettuccini. Sprinkle, if desired, with grated Parmesan cheese.

Conventional Directions: Increase wine to ½ cup. In large skillet, heat Italian dressing and cook green onions over medium heat 1 minute. Add assorted fresh vegetables, tomatoes and cook, stirring occasionally, 10 minutes or until vegetables are crisp-tender. Add wine, basil, seasoned salt and seasoned pepper and cook 2 minutes. Toss and sprinkle as above.

°***Assorted fresh vegetables:*** *Use any combination of the following to equal 2 quarts—asparagus cut into 2-inch pieces, broccoli florets, sliced carrots, yellow squash or zucchini.*

Nutrients per serving:			
Calories	275	Sodium	731 mg
Fat	3 g	Cholesterol	54 mg

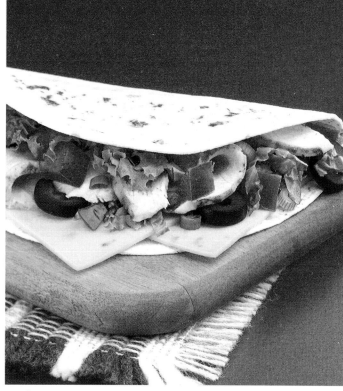

Jalapeño Chicken Fajitas

Jalapeño Chicken Fajitas

Low Cholesterol

Makes 8 fajitas

¼ cup ReaLime® Lime Juice from Concentrate
2 tablespoons water
1 clove garlic, chopped
8 ounces skinned boneless chicken breasts
8 (6-inch) flour tortillas, warmed
8 slices BORDEN® Lite-line® Jalapeño Flavor
   Process Cheese Product, cut in half
   diagonally°
   Garnishes: Salsa, shredded lettuce, green
   onions, chopped tomatoes, sliced ripe olives

In medium bowl, combine ReaLime® lime juice, water and garlic; add chicken. Marinate in refrigerator 3 to 4 hours. Remove chicken from marinade; grill or broil as desired. Place 2 Lite-line® halves on each tortilla. Slice chicken diagonally into thin strips; place on tortillas. Top with garnishes; fold tortillas. Serve immediately. Refrigerate leftovers.

°*"½ the calories" 8% milkfat version*

Nutrients per serving:			
Calories	161	Sodium	453 mg
Fat	4 g	Cholesterol	23 mg

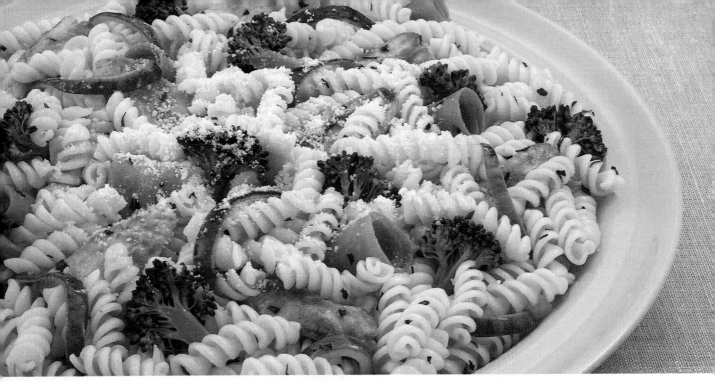

Rotini Stir-Fry

Rotini Stir-Fry

Low Sodium

Makes 8 servings

½ of a (1-pound) package CREAMETTE® Rotini, uncooked
2 tablespoons olive or vegetable oil
2 whole boneless skinless chicken breasts, cut into strips (about 12 ounces)
1 cup fresh broccoli flowerets
1 cup carrot curls
½ cup sliced red onion
¼ cup water
½ teaspoon WYLER'S® Chicken-Flavor Instant Bouillon
½ teaspoon tarragon leaves
2 tablespoons grated Parmesan cheese

Prepare CREAMETTE® Rotini as package directs; drain. In large skillet, heat oil; add chicken, broccoli, carrots and onion. Cook and stir over medium heat until broccoli is tender-crisp. Add water, bouillon and tarragon; cook and stir until chicken is cooked through. Add hot cooked rotini and Parmesan cheese; toss to coat. Serve immediately. Refrigerate leftovers.

Note: To reduce sodium, substitute low-sodium bouillon.

Nutrients per serving:			
Calories	225	Sodium	123 mg
Fat	6 g	Cholesterol	37 mg

Herb-Marinated Chicken Kabobs

Quick & Easy

Makes 4 servings

4 skinless boneless chicken breast halves
2 small zucchini, cut into ½-inch slices
1 large red bell pepper, cut into 1-inch squares
½ cup HEINZ® Wine Vinegar
½ cup tomato juice
2 tablespoons vegetable oil
1 tablespoon chopped sweet onion
1 tablespoon brown sugar
2 cloves garlic, minced
½ teaspoon dried oregano leaves, crushed
½ teaspoon pepper

Lightly flatten chicken breasts; cut each breast lengthwise into 3 strips. Place chicken in bowl with zucchini and bell pepper.

For marinade: Combine vinegar and remaining ingredients in jar. Cover; shake vigorously. Pour marinade over chicken and vegetables. Cover; marinate in refrigerator about 1 hour. Drain chicken and vegetables, reserving marinade. Alternately thread chicken and vegetables onto skewers; brush with marinade. Broil 3 to 5 inches from heat source, until chicken is cooked, about 8 to 10 minutes; turn and brush occasionally with marinade. Serve with rice, if desired.

Nutrients per serving:			
Calories	234	Sodium	189 mg
Fat	9 g	Cholesterol	68 mg

"Grilled" Tuna with Vegetables in Herb Butter

Quick & Easy

Makes 4 servings

4 pieces heavy-duty aluminum foil, each 12×18 inches
1 can (12½ ounces) STARKIST® Tuna, drained and broken into chunks
1 cup slivered red or green bell peppers
1 cup slivered yellow squash or zucchini
1 cup pea pods, cut crosswise into halves
1 cup slivered carrots
4 green onions, cut into 2-inch slices
3 tablespoons butter or margarine, melted
1 tablespoon lemon or lime juice
1 clove garlic, minced
2 teaspoons dried tarragon, crushed
1 teaspoon dill weed
  Salt and pepper to taste (optional)

On each piece of foil mound tuna, bell peppers, squash, pea pods, carrots and onions.

For herb butter: In a small bowl stir together butter, lemon juice, garlic, tarragon and dill weed. Drizzle over tuna and vegetables. Sprinkle with salt and pepper. Fold edges of each foil square together to make packets.

To grill: Place foil packets about 4 inches above hot coals. Grill for 10 to 12 minutes, or until heated through, turning packet over halfway through grill time.

To bake: Place foil packets on a baking sheet. Bake in preheated 450°F oven for 15 to 20 minutes, or until heated through.

To serve: Cut an "x" on top of each packet; peel back the foil.

Nutrients per serving:

Calories	235	Sodium	519 mg
Fat	9 g	Cholesterol	70 mg

Spaghetti Pizza Deluxe

Makes 8 servings

1 package (7 ounces) CREAMETTE® Spaghetti, uncooked
½ cup skim milk
1 egg, beaten
  Vegetable cooking spray
½ pound lean ground beef
1 medium onion, chopped
1 medium green bell pepper, chopped
2 cloves garlic, minced
1 can (15 ounces) tomato sauce
1 teaspoon Italian seasoning
1 teaspoon any salt-free herb seasoning
¼ teaspoon pepper
2 cups sliced fresh mushrooms
2 cups shredded part-skim mozzarella cheese

Prepare CREAMETTE® Spaghetti as package directs; drain. In medium bowl, blend milk and egg; add spaghetti and toss to coat. Spray 15×10-inch jellyroll pan with vegetable cooking spray. Spread spaghetti mixture evenly in prepared pan. In large skillet, cook beef, onion, green pepper and garlic until beef is no longer pink; drain. Add tomato sauce and seasonings; simmer 5 minutes. Spoon meat mixture evenly over spaghetti. Top with mushrooms and cheese. Bake in 350° oven for 20 minutes. Let stand 5 minutes before cutting. Refrigerate leftovers.

Note: To reduce sodium, substitute no-salt added tomato sauce.

Nutrients per serving:

Calories	267	Sodium	499 mg
Fat	9 g	Cholesterol	76 mg

Spaghetti Pizza Deluxe

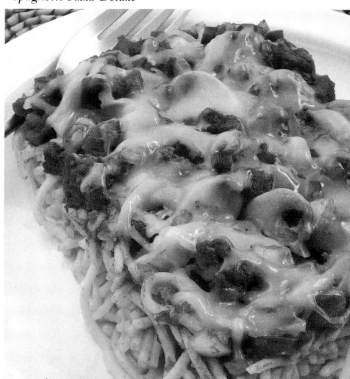

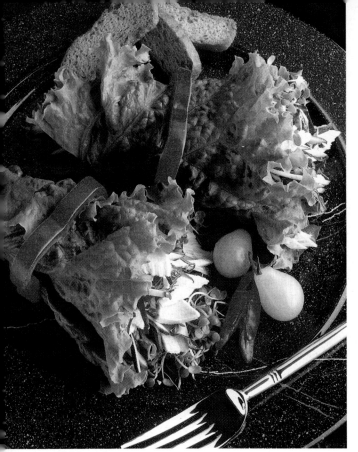

Tuna-Lettuce Bundles

Tuna-Lettuce Bundles

Quick & Easy

Makes 1 serving

2 large leaves leaf lettuce
1 can (3¼ ounces) STARKIST® Tuna, drained and
    broken into small chunks
½ cup shredded red cabbage
¼ cup shredded zucchini
¼ cup alfalfa sprouts
1 tablespoon reduced-calorie thousand island or
    blue cheese dressing
    Pepper to taste
2 red or green bell pepper rings

Trim stalks from lettuce leaves. In a small bowl toss
together tuna, cabbage, zucchini and sprouts. Stir in
dressing; season to taste with pepper. Spoon ½ of the
salad mixture in center of each leaf. Roll up leaves,
enclosing filling. Secure lettuce bundles by slipping a
bell pepper ring over each. Place bundles seam side
down on plate.

Nutrients per serving:

Calories	190	Sodium	570 mg
Fat	2 g	Cholesterol	43 mg

Linguine with White Clam Sauce

Low Cholesterol

Makes 8 servings

1 package (1 pound) CREAMETTE® Linguine,
    uncooked
2 tablespoons olive or vegetable oil
2 cloves garlic, minced
2 (6½-ounce *each*) cans SNOW'S® or DOXSEE®
    Chopped Clams, drain and reserve liquid
½ cup chopped parsley
¼ cup dry white wine
1 teaspoon basil leaves

Prepare CREAMETTE® linguine as package directs;
drain. In medium skillet, heat oil and garlic. Stir in
reserved clam liquid and parsley; cook and stir 3
minutes. Add clams, wine and basil. Simmer 5
minutes. Toss clam sauce with hot cooked linguine.
Serve immediately. Refrigerate leftovers.

Nutrients per serving:

Calories	293	Sodium	232 mg
Fat	5 g	Cholesterol	15 mg

Beef Cubed Steaks Provençale

Low Sodium

Makes 4 servings

4 lean beef cubed steaks (about 4 ounces each)
2 cloves garlic, minced
½ teaspoon dried basil leaves
¼ teaspoon pepper
1½ teaspoons olive oil
2 small zucchini, thinly sliced
6 cherry tomatoes, cut in half
1½ teaspoons grated Parmesan cheese
    Salt (optional)

Combine garlic, basil and pepper; divide mixture in
half. Press half of seasoning mixture evenly into both
sides of beef cubed steaks; reserve. Heat oil and
remaining seasoning mixture in large nonstick skillet
over medium heat. Add zucchini; cook and stir 3
minutes. Add tomatoes; continue cooking 1 minute,
stirring frequently. Remove vegetables to platter;
sprinkle with cheese and keep warm. Increase heat to
medium-high. Add 2 of the steaks to same pan;
panbroil to desired doneness, 3 to 4 minutes, turning
once. Repeat with remaining 2 steaks. Season steaks
with salt, if desired. Serve with reserved vegetables;
garnish as desired.

Nutrients per serving:

Calories	223	Sodium	60 mg
Fat	10 g	Cholesterol	81 mg

Favorite recipe from **National Livestock and Meat Board**

Herb-Marinated Chuck Steak

Makes 4 servings

1 pound boneless beef chuck shoulder steak, cut
   1-inch thick
¼ cup chopped onion
2 tablespoons *each* chopped parsley and white
   vinegar
1 tablespoon vegetable oil
2 teaspoons Dijon-style mustard
1 clove garlic, minced
½ teaspoon dried thyme leaves

Combine onion, parsley, vinegar, oil, mustard, garlic
and thyme. Place beef chuck shoulder steak in plastic
bag; add onion mixture, spreading evenly over both
sides. Close bag securely; marinate in refrigerator 6 to
8 hours (or overnight, if desired), turning at least
once. Pour off marinade; discard. Place steak on rack
in broiler pan so surface of meat is 3 to 5 inches from
heat source. Broil about 16 minutes for rare and
about 18 minutes for medium, turning once. Carve
steak diagonally across the grain into thin slices.
Garnish as desired.

Nutrients per serving:

Calories	216	Sodium	94 mg
Fat	10 g	Cholesterol	85 mg

Favorite recipe from **National Livestock and Meat Board**

Oven Crisped Fish

Makes 4 servings

½ cup unseasoned bread crumbs
2 tablespoons grated Parmesan cheese
2 teaspoons grated lemon peel
¾ teaspoon marjoram
½ teaspoon paprika
¼ teaspoon dried thyme leaves
⅛ teaspoon garlic powder
1 pound cod fillets
3 tablespoons lemon juice
2 tablespoons white wine
2 tablespoons PURITAN® Oil

Heat oven to 425°F. Oil 13×9×2-inch pan. Combine
bread crumbs and next 6 ingredients. Set aside. Rinse
fillets. Pat dry. Combine lemon juice and wine in
shallow pan. Dip each fillet in lemon mixture, then in
seasoned crumbs. Make certain each piece is well
coated. Place fish in pan. Drizzle evenly with
PURITAN® Oil. Bake at 425°F for 20 to 25 minutes
or until fish flakes easily when tested with fork. Cut
into serving size pieces, if desired.

Nutrients per serving:

Calories	220	Sodium	210 mg
Fat	9 g	Cholesterol	60 mg

Herb-Marinated Chuck Steak

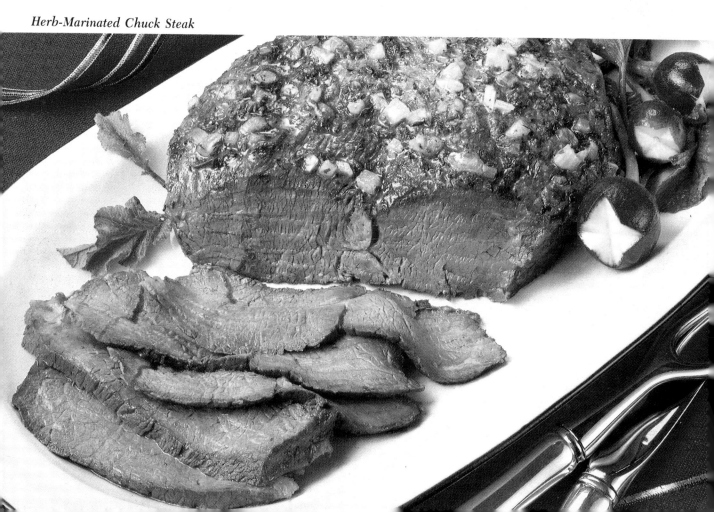

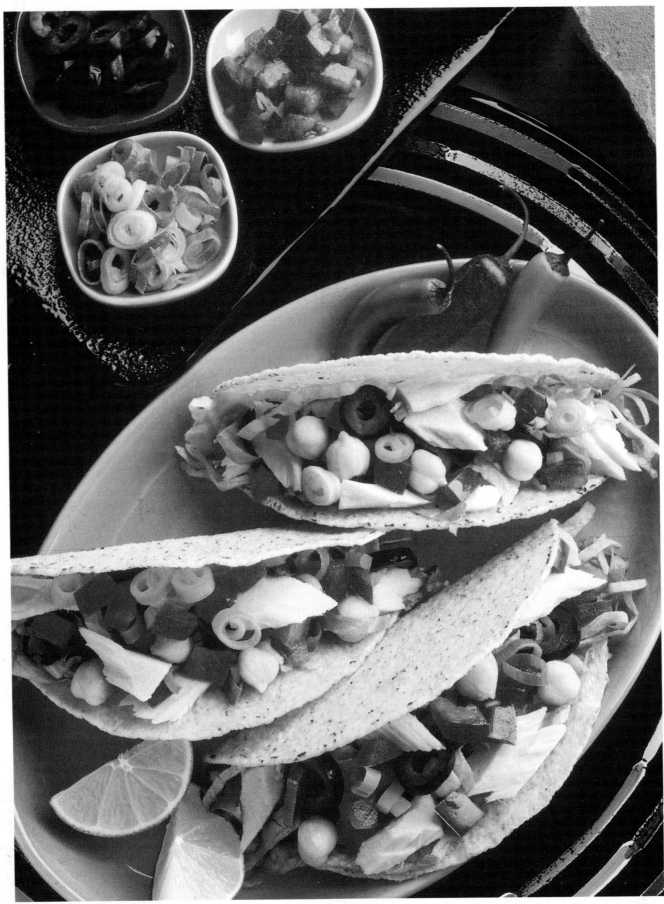

Tuna Tacos

Tuna Tacos

Low Cholesterol

Makes 4 servings

1 can (6½ ounces) STARKIST® Tuna, drained and flaked
⅓ cup chopped green onions
¼ cup bottled salsa
2 cups shredded lettuce
8 corn taco shells°
1 cup garbanzo beans
1 cup chopped tomatoes
⅓ cup sliced pitted ripe olives
   Salsa, shredded low-fat cheese, diced avocado, chopped green chilies for toppings (optional)

In a medium bowl toss together tuna, onions and salsa until combined. To assemble tacos: Sprinkle lettuce into each taco shell. Divide tuna mixture among tacos, along with garbanzo beans, tomatoes and olives. Garnish as desired with toppings.

°Substitute 8 (6-inch) flour tortillas for the taco shells if soft tacos are preferred.

Nutrients per serving (2 tacos):			
Calories:	273	Sodium	418 mg
Fat	4 g	Cholesterol	37 mg

Chicken Mushroom Crepes

Makes 4 servings

Crepes

3 tablespoons uncooked rolled oats
5 egg whites
1 tablespoon finely chopped onion
1 tablespoon chopped green onion
1 tablespoon finely chopped spinach
½ teaspoon salt
½ teaspoon vanilla (optional)
2 packets Equal™

In a small skillet over high heat, lightly toast the oats, shaking the pan almost constantly until they're light brown. Place all crepe ingredients except the Equal™ in blender. Process well, add Equal™ and blend again. Heat a 10-inch Teflon skillet until very hot. Pour ¼ crepe batter into pan, tip the pan quickly to coat the bottom with crepe batter and cook about 1 minute, or until edges begin to curl away from pan. Turn crepe out onto dish and repeat process 3 more times, blending batter until frothy each time. Set aside.

Chicken Filling

1 package (12 ounces) low-fat cottage cheese
1 cup plus 2 tablespoons defatted chicken stock, in all
2 teaspoons arrowroot
1 tablespoon Chef Paul Prudhomme's POULTRY MAGIC®, in all
8 ounces skinless boneless chicken breasts, cut into short strips
½ cup chopped onion
¼ cup chopped green bell pepper
½ teaspoon minced fresh garlic
3 cups thinly sliced mushrooms (about 6 large)
½ cup diced yellow squash
½ cup diced zucchini

Make a mock cream by placing cottage cheese in blender and processing until very creamy, about 4 minutes. Add 3 tablespoons chicken stock and blend again until very smooth and creamy. Set aside. Combine arrowroot with 1 tablespoon stock and set aside.

Mix 1 teaspoon POULTRY MAGIC® into chicken, blending well until all chicken is evenly coated.

Place a 10-inch skillet over high heat. When pan is very hot, add seasoned chicken and quickly bronze, cooking approximately 2 minutes on each side. Remove from skillet. Let skillet get very hot again; add onion, bell pepper and 1 teaspoon POULTRY MAGIC® and cook 3 minutes, stirring once just to brown evenly and distribute the seasoning throughout the vegetables. Stir in 3 tablespoons stock and scrape up pan bottom. Cook 3 minutes and add 3 tablespoons stock around sides of pan and scrape. Cook 1½ minutes, and add minced garlic and mushrooms. Stir well and add squash and zucchini. Stir gently and continue cooking 1 minute. Add ½ teaspoon POULTRY MAGIC® and stir to coat vegetables with seasoning. If sides of pan are browning fast, move vegetables to edges and use their moisture to scrape up brown coating on sides. Cook 4 minutes, add chicken back to pan and the remaining ½ cup stock. Scrape up pan bottom and cook 4 minutes. Add the arrowroot mixture to pan. Cook 1 minute and add 1 cup of the mock cream. Bring to a simmer and turn off heat. Add ½ teaspoon POULTRY MAGIC®. Mix well. Place remaining ½ cup chicken mixture in each crepe, roll up and top with another ¼ cup of mixture.

Nutrients per serving:			
Calories	243	Sodium	1689 mg
Fat	4 g	Cholesterol	56 mg

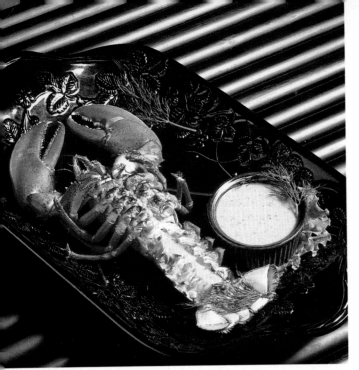

Spiced Broiled Lobster

Spiced Broiled Lobster

Quick & Easy

Makes 4 servings

4 Maine lobsters (1 to 1½ pounds *each*)
  Boiling water
½ cup WISH-BONE® Lite Italian Dressing
½ small onion, halved
1 tablespoon ketchup
1 tablespoon snipped fresh dill°
2 teaspoons Dijon-style mustard
⅛ teaspoon hot pepper sauce

Place each lobster on its stomach. With tip of sharp knife, make 2 deep criss-cross cuts in each lobster head. Immediately plunge into boiling water and boil 30 seconds or until lobster turns red. Remove from water; let cool slightly. Place each lobster on its back, then make lengthwise cut down each lobster tail; set aside.

In food processor or blender, process remaining ingredients; set aside.

In large shallow aluminum-foil-lined baking pan or on broiler rack, arrange prepared lobsters stomach side up, then brush tails with ⅓ of the dressing mixture. Broil on lower rack 20 minutes or until lobster meat turns opaque. (If lobsters brown too quickly, loosely cover with aluminum foil.) Serve with remaining dressing mixture for dipping.

°*Substitution: Use 1 teaspoon dried dill weed.*

Nutrients per serving:			
Calories	144	Sodium	1019 mg
Fat	1 g	Cholesterol	90 mg

Easy Tuna Melt

Quick & Easy

Makes 2 servings

1 can (3½ ounces) solid white water-pack tuna, drained
2 teaspoons reduced calorie salad dressing
1 teaspoon dill pickle relish
1 English muffin, split and toasted
2 tomato slices
2 slices BORDEN® Lite-line® Process Cheese Product, any flavor°

Combine tuna, salad dressing and relish. Top each muffin half with tomato slice then half of the tuna mixture and one Lite-line® slice. Broil or heat in microwave oven until Lite-line® slice begins to melt. Refrigerate leftovers.

°"½ the calories" 8% milkfat version

Nutrients per serving:			
Calories	186	Sodium	570 mg
Fat	6 g	Cholesterol	23 mg

Stir-Fry Beef & Noodles

Low Sodium

Makes 8 servings

2 tablespoons vegetable oil
½ pound beef flank steak, cut diagonally into thin slices
2 cups fresh broccoli flowerets
2 cups sliced fresh mushrooms
1 large onion, chopped
1 clove garlic, minced
2 tablespoons capers, drained
1 teaspoon WYLER'S® Beef-Flavor Instant Bouillon
¼ cup red wine or water
½ of a (1-pound) package CREAMETTE® Egg Noodles, uncooked

In large skillet, heat oil. Add beef; cook and stir just until tender; drain. Add broccoli, mushrooms, onion, garlic, capers and bouillon; cook and stir just until broccoli is tender-crisp. Add wine; cook 1 minute. Keep warm. Prepare CREAMETTE® Egg Noodles as package directs; drain. Serve meat mixture over hot cooked noodles. Refrigerate leftovers.

Note: To reduce sodium, substitute low-sodium bouillon.

Nutrients per serving:			
Calories	214	Sodium	136 mg
Fat	6 g	Cholesterol	29 mg

Saucy Pork and Peppers

Makes 4 servings

2 fresh limes
¼ cup 62%-less-sodium soy sauce
4 cloves garlic, crushed
1 teaspoon oregano leaves
½ teaspoon thyme leaves
    Dash cayenne pepper
2 to 3 fresh parsley sprigs
1 bay leaf
1 pound pork tenderloin, cut into 1-inch cubes
1 tablespoon olive oil
1 teaspoon brown sugar
2 medium onions, each cut into 8 pieces
2 medium tomatoes, each cut into 8 pieces and
    seeded
1 large red bell pepper, cut into 8 pieces
1 large green bell pepper, cut into 8 pieces

Remove peel from limes using vegetable peeler. Squeeze juice from limes. In small bowl, combine lime juice and peel, soy sauce, garlic, oregano leaves, thyme leaves, cayenne pepper, parsley and bay leaf; blend well. Place pork cubes in plastic bag or nonmetal bowl. Pour marinade mixture over pork, turning to coat. Seal bag or cover dish; marinate at least 2 hours or overnight in refrigerator, turning pork several times.

Remove lime peel, parsley sprigs and bay leaf from marinade; discard. Remove pork from marinade, reserving marinade. Drain pork well. Heat oil in large skillet over high heat. Add brown sugar; stir until sugar is brown and bubbly. Add pork cubes; cook and stir about 5 minutes or until pork is browned. Reduce heat to low. Add onions, tomatoes, peppers and reserved marinade; simmer 10 to 15 minutes or until pork is tender.

Nutrients per serving:

Calories	243	Sodium	547 mg
Fat	8 g	Cholesterol	79 mg

Favorite recipe from **National Pork Producers Council**

Turkey with Orange Sauce

Low Sodium

Makes 4 servings

2 turkey thighs or turkey drumsticks
    (2 to 3 pounds)°
½ teaspoon paprika
1 medium onion, sliced
½ cup thawed orange juice concentrate, undiluted
⅓ cup water
2 tablespoons brown sugar
2 tablespoons chopped parsley
2 teaspoons soy sauce
½ teaspoon ground ginger

Rinse turkey parts and pat dry. Place under broiler to brown. (If using only thigh, remove skin.) Remove to Dutch oven or roasting pan and sprinkle with paprika. Arrange onion slices over turkey parts. In small bowl, combine juice concentrate, water, brown sugar, parsley, soy sauce and ginger. Pour over turkey and onions.

Cover and bake approximately 1 hour in a 400°F preheated oven until turkey is tender, basting once or twice. Slice meat, coat with sauce and garnish with orange twists. Serve with rice or pasta.

°*Thighs may be boned before cooking*

Nutrients per serving:

Calories	152	Sodium	210 mg
Fat	5 g	Cholesterol	56 mg

Favorite recipe from **National Turkey Federation**

Saucy Pork and Peppers

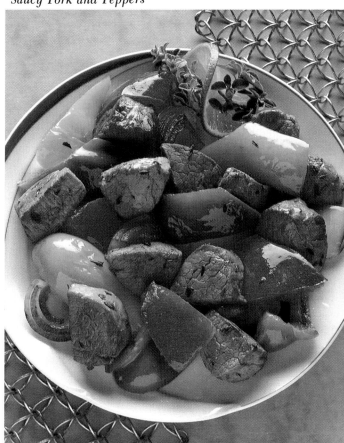

Barbecued Pork Chops

Low Sodium

Makes 6 servings

2 tablespoons PURITAN® Oil
6 loin pork chops, trimmed of excess fat
1 medium onion, chopped
3 cloves garlic, minced
1 can (6 ounces) no-salt-added tomato paste
½ cup cider vinegar
¼ cup plus 2 tablespoons firmly packed brown sugar
¼ cup water
3 tablespoons Worcestershire sauce
1 teaspoon dry mustard
1 teaspoon chili powder
¼ teaspoon pepper
¼ teaspoon salt

1. Heat oven to 350°F.

2. Heat PURITAN® Oil in large skillet over medium-high heat. Sauté pork chops until lightly browned. Remove chops from skillet. Place in 11×7-inch baking dish in single layer. Set aside.

3. Add onion and garlic to skillet. Cook over medium heat until soft. Stir in remaining ingredients. Simmer 5 minutes.

4. Pour sauce over chops. Turn to coat. Cover. Bake at 350°F for 45 to 60 minutes or until chops are tender.

Microwave Directions:
1. Combine PURITAN® Oil, onion, and garlic in 11×7-inch microwave-safe dish. Cover with plastic wrap. Microwave on High 3 minutes. Stir after 1 minute, 30 seconds.

2. Add remaining ingredients. Stir well. Place uncooked chops in sauce. Turn to coat. Cover. Microwave on High 16 minutes. Turn dish every 4 minutes. Rearrange chops after 8 minutes. Let stand 5 minutes, covered, before serving.

Nutrients per serving:			
Calories	200	Sodium	90 mg
Fat	10 g	Cholesterol	70 mg

Shrimp Creole

Quick & Easy

Makes 4 servings

1 can (14½ ounces) whole peeled tomatoes, undrained and chopped
½ cup WISH-BONE® Lite Italian Dressing
1 medium green pepper, cut into chunks
1 medium onion, sliced
1 pound uncooked medium shrimp, cleaned
⅛ teaspoon crushed red pepper
2 cups hot cooked rice

Discard ½ cup liquid from tomatoes. In 1½-quart microwave-safe casserole, microwave Italian dressing, green pepper and onion, covered, at High (full power) 4 minutes or until tender, stirring once. Add tomatoes with remaining liquid and microwave covered at High 5 minutes. Add shrimp and red pepper and microwave, covered, at High 3 minutes or until shrimp turn pink, stirring once. To serve: Arrange shrimp mixture over hot rice.

Conventional Directions: In medium skillet, heat Italian dressing and cook green pepper and onion over medium heat, stirring occasionally, 5 minutes or until tender. Stir in tomatoes with liquid and simmer covered 15 minutes. Add shrimp and red pepper and simmer covered an additional 5 minutes or until shrimp turn pink. Serve as above.

Nutrients per serving:			
Calories	274	Sodium	727 mg
Fat	2 g	Cholesterol	140 mg

Shrimp Creole

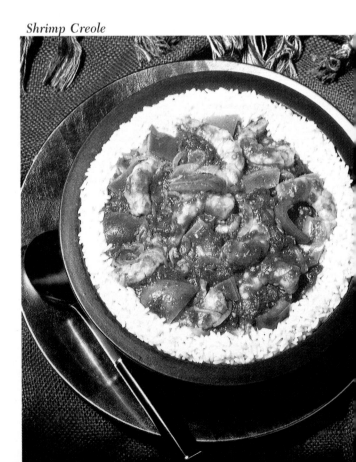

Pizza Stuffed Peppers

Quick & Easy

Makes 4 servings

½ pound ground round
¼ cup finely chopped onion
4 slices BORDEN® Lite-line® Process Cheese
  ' Product (any flavor), cut into small pieces°
½ cup prepared pizza sauce
¼ teaspoon Italian seasoning
2 medium green bell peppers, halved, seeded and
  blanched

Preheat oven to 350°. In medium skillet, brown meat
and onion; drain. Add remaining ingredients except
peppers. Cook and stir until Lite-line® pieces melt.
Arrange peppers in shallow baking dish; spoon
mixture into peppers. Bake 10 to 15 minutes or until
hot. Refrigerate leftovers.

°"½ the calories" 8% milkfat version

Nutrients per serving:

Calories	192	Sodium	484 mg
Fat	8 g	Cholesterol	58 mg

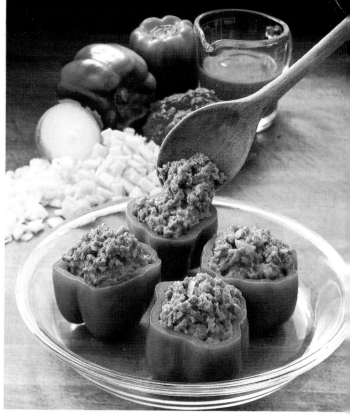

Pizza Stuffed Peppers

Light and Easy Turkey Tenderloin

Low Sodium

Makes 2 servings

½ cup julienne sliced carrots
1 turkey breast tenderloin (about ½ pound)
2 green onions, sliced
2 slices red or green bell pepper
⅛ teaspoon garlic powder
⅛ teaspoon dried rosemary leaves, crushed
⅛ teaspoon salt
  Dash pepper
1 tablespoon white wine

1. Preheat oven to 400°F.

2. On a 12×16-inch foil rectangle, place carrots; top
with tenderloin. Arrange onions and pepper slices
over tenderloin. Sprinkle with garlic powder,
rosemary, salt and pepper.

3. Fold edges of foil up to form a bowl shape. Pour
wine over ingredients. Bring two opposite foil sides
together; fold edges over and down to seal. Fold short
ends up and over.

4. On a small cookie sheet, place foil bundle and bake
20 to 25 minutes or until meat reaches 170°F. Check
for doneness by opening foil bundle carefully to insert
meat thermometer in thickest part of meat.

Nutrients per serving:

Calories	150	Sodium	226 mg
Fat	2 g	Cholesterol	70 mg

Favorite recipe from **National Turkey Federation**

Greek Lamb Sauté with Mostaccioli

Low Sodium

Makes 8 servings

½ of a (1-pound) package CREAMETTE®
  Mostaccioli, uncooked
1 tablespoon olive or vegetable oil
1 medium green bell pepper, chopped
1 medium onion, chopped
1 medium eggplant, peeled, seeded and cut into
  1-inch cubes
2 cloves garlic, minced
½ pound lean boneless lamb, cut into ¾-inch
  cubes
2 fresh tomatoes, peeled, seeded and chopped
¼ teaspoon ground nutmeg
¼ cup grated Parmesan cheese

Prepare CREAMETTE® Mostaccioli as package
directs; drain. In large skillet, heat oil; add green
pepper, onion, eggplant and garlic. Cook and stir until
tender-crisp. Add lamb; cook until tender. Stir in
tomatoes and nutmeg; heat through. Toss meat
mixture with hot cooked mostaccioli and Parmesan
cheese. Serve immediately. Refrigerate leftovers.

Nutrients per serving:

Calories	205	Sodium	82 mg
Fat	5 g	Cholesterol	29 mg

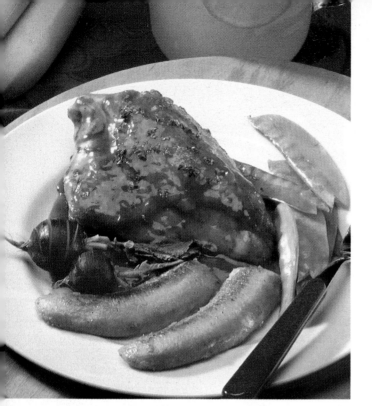

Chicken Columbia

Chicken Columbia

Low Sodium

Makes 4 servings

2 green-tip, medium DOLE® Bananas, peeled
2 tablespoons vegetable oil, divided
2 whole chicken breasts, split, boned
2 cloves garlic, minced
2 tablespoons minced gingerroot
  Orange peel strips°
½ cup orange juice
½ cup water, divided
2 tablespoons chopped chutney
2 teaspoons cornstarch

Cut bananas in half crosswise, then lengthwise. Sauté bananas in one tablespoon oil 30 to 45 seconds, shaking skillet. Remove from skillet. Add one more tablespoon oil to skillet. Brown chicken on both sides in hot oil. Add garlic and gingerroot; sauté. Stir in orange peel and juice, ¼ cup water and chutney. Cover, simmer 20 minutes. Mix cornstarch and remaining ¼ cup water; stir into pan juices. Cook until sauce boils and thickens. Top chicken with bananas. Generously spoon sauce over all.

°*Use vegetable peeler to cut thin strips from orange.*

Nutrients per serving:			
Calories	292	Sodium	79 mg
Fat	9 g	Cholesterol	68 mg

Pork Curry

Quick & Easy

Makes 4 servings

1 tablespoon vegetable oil
1 pound pork tenderloin, cut into ½-inch cubes
¾ cup coarsely chopped onion
⅓ cup chopped celery
1 medium tomato, seeded and chopped
1½ cups chopped apple, unpared
1 cup water
4 tablespoons golden raisins
3 tablespoons curry powder
1 teaspoon instant chicken bouillon granules
⅛ teaspoon garlic powder
  Hot cooked rice (optional)
  Plain yogurt (optional)
4 tablespoons chopped peanuts (optional)

In a large frying pan heat oil to medium-hot. Add pork cubes, onion and celery. Cook, stirring occasionally, until pork is brown and vegetables are tender. Stir in tomato, apple, water, raisins, curry powder, bouillon granules and garlic powder; mix well. Reduce temperature to low. Cover and cook, stirring occasionally, 10 minutes. Remove cover and continue cooking 5 to 10 minutes, until of desired consistency. Serve on a bed of hot cooked rice and top each serving with plain yogurt and chopped peanuts, if desired.

Nutrients per serving:			
Calories	243	Sodium	311 mg
Fat	7 g	Cholesterol	73 mg

Favorite recipe from **National Pork Producers Council**

Pork Curry

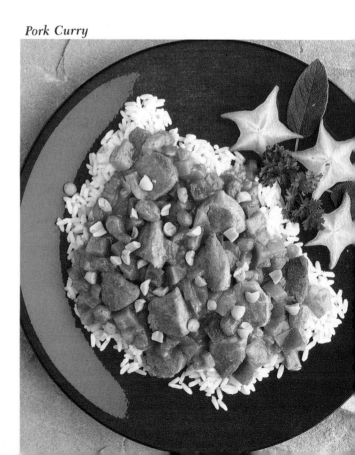

Ham Breakfast Sandwich

Low Cholesterol

Makes 3 sandwiches

1 ounce Neufchatel or light cream cheese,
   softened
2 teaspoons apricot spreadable fruit
2 teaspoons plain nonfat yogurt
6 slices raisin bread
   Lettuce leaves
1 package (6 ounces) ECKRICH® Lite Lower Salt
   Ham
3 Granny Smith apple rings

Combine cheese, spreadable fruit and yogurt in small
bowl. Spread on bread. To make each sandwich: Place
lettuce on 1 slice bread. Top with 2 slices ham, 1
apple ring and another slice of bread.

Nutrients per serving:			
Calories	223	Sodium	963 mg
Fat	5 g	Cholesterol	5 mg

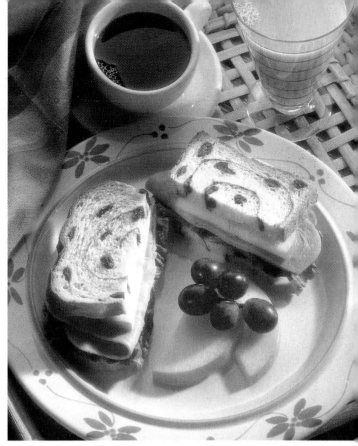

Ham Breakfast Sandwich

Butterflied Eye Round Roast

Low Sodium

Makes 12 servings

1 beef eye round roast (3 pounds)
¼ cup *each* red wine vinegar and water
2 tablespoons olive oil
2 cloves garlic, minced
1 tablespoon chopped fresh thyme *or* 1 teaspoon
   dried thyme leaves
½ teaspoon crushed red pepper

Butterfly beef eye round roast by cutting horizontally
through the center (parallel to surface of meat), the
length and width of roast. Do not cut through
opposite side of roast. Open meat and lay flat.
Combine vinegar, water, oil, garlic, thyme and red
pepper. Place beef roast in plastic bag; add vinegar
mixture, turning to coat roast. Close bag securely;
marinate in refrigerator 6 to 8 hours (or overnight, if
desired), turning occasionally. Remove roast from
marinade; reserve marinade. Place beef on rack in
broiler pan so surface of meat is 5 to 7 inches from
heat source. Broil 20 to 25 minutes to desired
doneness (rare or medium), turning and basting with
reserved marinade occasionally. Tent with foil and
allow roast to stand 10 to 15 minutes in warm place
before carving. Carve roast into thin slices.

*Note: A beef eye round roast will yield four 3-ounce
cooked servings per pound.*

Nutrients per serving (3 ounces cooked beef):			
Calories	172	Sodium	53 mg
Fat	7 g	Cholesterol	59 mg

Favorite recipe from **National Livestock and Meat Board**

Light 'n' Saucy Shrimp

Low Sodium

Makes 3 to 4 servings

1 cup chopped onions
¼ cup chopped green bell pepper
2 cloves garlic, minced
¼ cup water
1 teaspoon granulated sugar
¼ teaspoon fines herbes
⅛ teaspoon pepper
1 can (14½ ounces) stewed tomatoes (no added
   salt), cut into bite-size pieces
¼ cup HEINZ® Apple Cider Vinegar
¾ pound medium-size raw shrimp, peeled,
   deveined
½ teaspoon cornstarch
½ teaspoon water
2 cups hot cooked rice

In 2-quart saucepan, combine first 7 ingredients;
simmer, covered, 10 minutes or until onions are
tender. Stir in tomatoes and vinegar; simmer, covered,
15 minutes, stirring occasionally. Add shrimp; simmer
an additional 5 minutes or until shrimp are cooked,
stirring occasionally. In small cup stir together
cornstarch and water. Thicken sauce with cornstarch
water mixture. Serve over rice.

Nutrients per serving:			
Calories	233	Sodium	54 mg
Fat	2 g	Cholesterol	173 mg

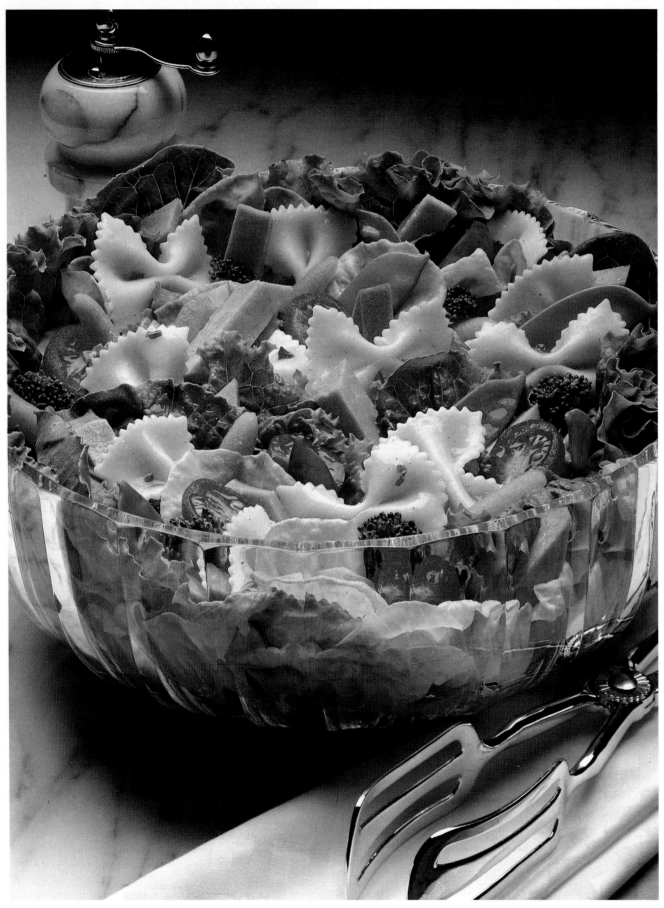

Zesty Pasta Salad

Salads & Side Dishes

Zesty Pasta Salad

Quick & Easy

Makes 6 servings

2 cups (8 ounces) ARMOUR® Lower Salt Ham, cut into julienne strips
2 cups pasta bowties or shells, cooked according to package directions omitting salt, drained
8 ounces California-blend frozen vegetables, thawed
5 cherry tomatoes, cut in half
¾ cup bottled low sodium, reduced calorie zesty Italian salad dressing
4 cups mixed greens, washed and drained

Combine ham, pasta, vegetables, tomatoes and salad dressing in large bowl; toss to coat well. Cover; refrigerate at least 1 hour before serving to blend flavors. To serve, arrange pasta mixture in lettuce-lined bowl or on platter.

Nutrients per serving:			
Calories	233	Sodium	344 mg
Fat	3 g	Cholesterol	19 mg

Cucumbers and Onions

Quick & Easy

Makes 6 servings

1 medium cucumber, thinly sliced
1 small onion, thinly sliced
1 can (5 fluid ounces) PET® Light Evaporated Skimmed Milk
¼ cup vinegar
1 teaspoon salt
1 teaspoon dried dill weed

In a medium bowl, combine cucumber and onion. In small bowl, combine remaining ingredients and pour over cucumber and onion; toss well. Chill before serving.

Nutrients per serving:			
Calories	33	Sodium	389 mg
Fat	1 g	Cholesterol	1 mg

Yogurt Dressing

Low Cholesterol

Makes 2 cups

2 cups plain lowfat yogurt
4 teaspoons chopped fresh mint *or* ¼ teaspoon dried dill weed
⅛ teaspoon TABASCO® pepper sauce

In small bowl combine yogurt, mint and TABASCO® pepper sauce; mix well. Cover; refrigerate.

Nutrients per serving (1 tablespoon):			
Calories	10	Sodium	10 mg
Fat	0 g	Cholesterol	0 mg

Red, Green & Gold Squash Platter

Low Cholesterol

Makes 8 servings

1 pound red bell peppers (3 medium)
2 tablespoons olive oil
¼ teaspoon grated lemon peel
1 tablespoon lemon juice
½ teaspoon dill weed
   Salt and pepper to taste
3 cups *each* sliced zucchini and crookneck squash
⅓ cup BLUE DIAMOND® Sliced Natural Almonds, toasted

Core and quarter red bell peppers. Place in single layer in glass baking dish. Cover; microwave at High power for 10 minutes. Process peppers and remaining ingredients except squash and almonds in blender or food processor until smooth. Place squash in 9×9-inch square glass baking dish. Cover; microwave at High power 3 to 4 minutes, until tender-crisp. Spoon squash onto serving platter. Toss with almonds. Drizzle with red pepper sauce to serve.

Nutrients per serving:			
Calories	84	Sodium	140 mg
Fat	6 g	Cholesterol	0 mg

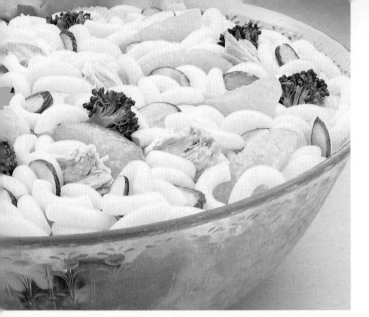

Creamettes® Chicken Salad

Creamettes® Chicken Salad

Low Sodium

Makes 8 servings

1 (7-ounce) package CREAMETTES® Elbow
    Macaroni (2 cups uncooked)
2 cups cubed cooked chicken or turkey (white
    meat)
2 cups fresh broccoli flowerets
4 medium oranges, peeled, sectioned and seeded
1 cup orange juice
¼ cup cider vinegar
1 teaspoon ground ginger
½ teaspoon paprika
¼ cup toasted sliced almonds

Prepare CREAMETTES® Elbow Macaroni as
package directs; drain. In large bowl, combine
macaroni, chicken, broccoli and oranges. In small
bowl, blend orange juice, vinegar, ginger and paprika;
toss with macaroni mixture. Cover; chill thoroughly.
Stir before serving. Garnish with almonds. Refrigerate
leftovers.

Nutrients per serving:			
Calories	222	Sodium	38 mg
Fat	4 g	Cholesterol	36 mg

Wild Rice Sauté

Low Cholesterol

Makes 6 servings

½ cup sliced, fresh mushrooms
¼ cup chopped green onions
1 clove garlic, minced
2 tablespoons HOLLYWOOD® Safflower Oil
3 cups cooked wild rice
¼ teaspoon salt
¼ teaspoon ground black pepper
¼ teaspoon dried rosemary sprigs
2 tablespoons peach schnapps liqueur

In a large skillet, sauté mushrooms, onions and garlic
in hot oil for 1½ minutes. Add rice, seasonings and
peach schnapps and cook 1½ minutes longer; stirring
frequently.

Nutrients per serving:			
Calories	143	Sodium	97 mg
Fat	5 g	Cholesterol	0 mg

Light Pasta Salad

Low Cholesterol

Makes 4 servings

½ cup MIRACLE WHIP® Light Reduced Calorie
    Salad Dressing with no cholesterol
½ cup KRAFT® "Zesty" Italian Reduced Calorie
    Dressing
2 cups (6 ounces) corkscrew noodles, cooked,
    drained
1 cup broccoli flowerets, partially-cooked
½ cup chopped green pepper
½ cup chopped tomato
¼ cup green onion slices

Combine dressings; mix well. Add remaining
ingredients; mix lightly. Chill. Serve with freshly
ground black pepper, if desired.

Nutrients per serving:			
Calories	260	Sodium	450 mg
Fat	9 g	Cholesterol	0 mg

Vegetable-Bulgur Salad

Low Cholesterol

Makes 1½ cups or 2 side-dish servings

⅓ cup bulgur wheat
1 cup hot water
1 teaspoon vegetable oil
¼ cup chopped sweet red pepper
¼ cup chopped zucchini
¾ cup V8 vegetable juice
1 teaspoon lemon juice
¼ teaspoon dried basil leaves, crushed
   Lettuce leaves (optional)
2 tablespoons chopped green onion for garnish

1. In 2-cup measure, stir together bulgur and hot water. Let stand 5 minutes; drain.

2. Meanwhile, in 6-inch skillet over medium heat, in hot oil, cook red pepper and zucchini until tender-crisp, stirring often.

3. Stir in V8 juice, lemon juice, basil and drained bulgur. Heat to boiling; reduce heat to low. Cover; simmer 15 minutes or until liquid is absorbed, stirring occasionally.

4. Serve warm or chilled. To serve chilled: Cover; refrigerate until serving time, at least 2 hours. Spoon into lettuce-lined salad bowl. Garnish with green onion.

Nutrients per serving:			
Calories	125	Sodium	289 mg
Fat	3 g	Cholesterol	0 mg

Vegetable-Bulgur Salad

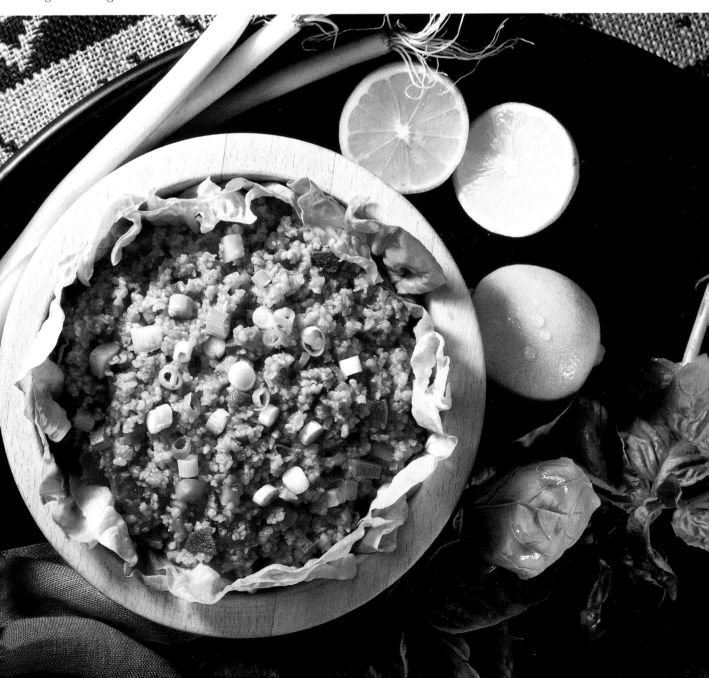

Bombay Banana Salad

Makes 4 servings

2 DOLE® Oranges
2 firm DOLE® Bananas, peeled, sliced
1 cup seedless red DOLE® Grapes
¼ cup DOLE® Whole Almonds, toasted
1 ripe DOLE® Banana, peeled
12 DOLE® Pitted Dates, halved

Dressing
½ cup dairy sour cream
1 tablespoon brown sugar or honey
1 tablespoon chopped chutney
½ teaspoon curry powder

Grate peel from 1 orange, reserve peel for dressing. Peel and slice oranges. In bowl, toss salad ingredients with dressing.

Dressing: Combine all ingredients in blender or food processor. Blend until smooth. Stir in grated orange peel.

Nutrients per serving:

Calories	240	Sodium	13 mg
Fat	9 g	Cholesterol	9 mg

Bombay Banana Salad

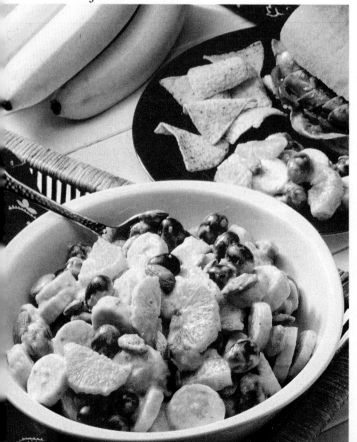

Thousand Island Dressing

Makes about 2 cups

⅔ cup PET® Light Evaporated Skimmed Milk
⅔ cup bottled chili sauce
⅔ cup safflower oil
¼ cup sweet pickle relish
1 tablespoon lemon juice
1 tablespoon sugar
1 teaspoon salt
⅛ teaspoon ground black pepper

Using a wire whisk combine all ingredients in a small bowl. Refrigerate until well chilled. Serve over tossed green salad.

Nutrients per serving (1 tablespoon):

Calories	54	Sodium	129 mg
Fat	5 g	Cholesterol	0 mg

Confetti Rice Salad

Makes 6 servings

2 chicken flavored bouillon cubes
1 cup long grain white rice
1 can (16 ounces) California cling peach slices in juice or extra light syrup
3 tablespoons tarragon-flavored white wine vinegar
1 tablespoon Dijon-style mustard
1 tablespoon olive oil
¼ teaspoon tarragon
1 cup chopped red peppers
½ cup frozen peas, thawed
⅓ cup raisins
¼ cup sliced green onions

In medium saucepan, combine bouillon cubes and 2 cups water; bring mixture to a boil. Stir in rice. Cover and simmer 20 minutes, until liquid is absorbed and rice is tender. Remove from heat; cool 5 minutes. Drain peaches, reserving ¼ cup liquid. Save remainder for other uses. Cut peach slices in half and set aside. Mix reserved peach liquid with vinegar, mustard, olive oil and tarragon. Stir into cooled rice; add remaining ingredients *except* reserved peaches. Cool completely, tossing occasionally. Stir in reserved peaches and chill before serving.

Nutrients per serving:

Calories	210	Sodium	317 mg
Fat	3 g	Cholesterol	.33 mg

Favorite recipe from **California Cling Peach Advisory Board**

Warm Turkey Salad

Makes 2 servings

1 medium DOLE® Fresh Pineapple
4 ounces green beans or broccoli, steamed
2 carrots, slivered or sliced
½ cup slivered jicama or radishes
½ cup slivered red bell pepper
  Crisp salad greens
  Salt and pepper to taste
2 turkey cutlets (½ pound)
1 tablespoon vegetable oil
  Lite Honey Mustard Dressing (recipe follows)

Twist crown from pineapple. Cut pineapple in half lengthwise. Refrigerate half for another use, such as fruit salads. Cut remaining half in half lengthwise. Remove fruit from shells with knife. Cut each quarter into 4 spears. Arrange pineapple, green beans, carrots, jicama and red bell pepper on 2 dinner plates lined with crisp salad greens, leaving space for sautéed turkey. Lightly salt and pepper turkey. In medium skillet, brown turkey on both sides in oil. Cover, simmer 5 to 7 minutes. Add 1 tablespoon water if needed. Remove from skillet. Cut turkey crosswise into 4 or 5 slices. Arrange on salad plates with pineapple and vegetables. Serve with Lite Honey Mustard Dressing.

Lite Honey Mustard Dressing:

¼ cup cholesterol free reduced calorie mayonnaise
1 to 2 tablespoons pineapple juice or orange juice
1 teaspoon honey
1 teaspoon Dijon-style mustard
¼ teaspoon tarragon, crumbled

Combine all ingredients.

Nutrients per serving:			
Calories	286	Sodium	233 mg
Fat	10 g	Cholesterol	30 mg

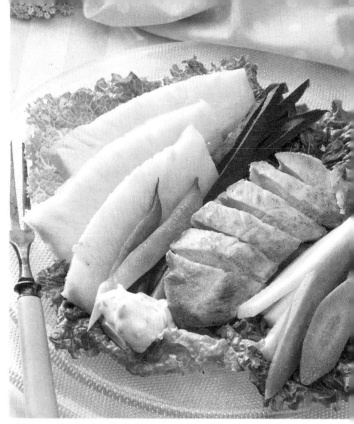

Warm Turkey Salad

Holiday Stir-Fry

Makes 4 servings

¾ teaspoon finely chopped fresh jalapeño, or to taste
1 clove garlic, minced
2 tablespoons HOLLYWOOD® Peanut or Safflower Oil
20 fresh green beans, ends trimmed
3 cups fresh spinach, washed and trimmed
2 cups finely shredded red cabbage
⅓ cup chopped red pepper
¾ cup sliced mushrooms

In a large skillet, cook jalapeño and garlic in hot oil for 30 seconds. Add green beans and stir-fry for 1 minute. Cover and cook an additional 2½ minutes. Add remaining ingredients except mushrooms and stir-fry for 2 minutes. Add mushrooms and stir-fry an additional 1½ minutes. Serve hot.

Nutrients per serving:			
Calories	89	Sodium	36 mg
Fat	7 g	Cholesterol	0 mg

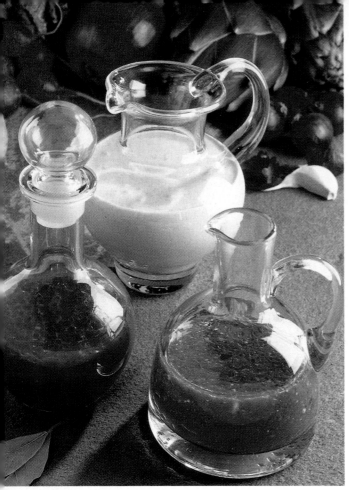

Clockwise from top: Creamy V8 Dressing, Ginger-Soy Dressing, Rosy Blue Cheese Dressing

Creamy V8 Dressing

Low Sodium

Makes 2½ cups

1 package (8 ounces) Neufchatel or reduced-calorie cream cheese, softened
1 cup reduced-calorie mayonnaise
1 cup V8 vegetable juice
3 cloves garlic, minced
1 teaspoon lemon juice

In medium bowl, blend Neufchatel until smooth. Gradually stir in mayonnaise until well blended. Stir in V8 juice, garlic and lemon juice. Cover; refrigerate until serving time, at least 2 hours. Use as a salad dressing, for dipping or as a sandwich spread.

Nutrients per serving (1 tablespoon):

Calories	32	Sodium	74 mg
Fat	3 g	Cholesterol	6 mg

Rosy Blue Cheese Dressing

Low Sodium

Makes 1 cup

¾ cup V8 vegetable juice
3 tablespoons vegetable oil
2 tablespoons crumbled blue cheese
1 tablespoon lemon juice
1 tablespoon finely chopped onion
1 clove garlic, minced

In covered jar, combine all ingredients. Shake until well blended. Cover; refrigerate until serving time, at least 2 hours. Shake again before using. Serve over salad greens or vegetable salads.

Nutrients per serving (1 tablespoon):

Calories	29	Sodium	50 mg
Fat	3 g	Cholesterol	1 mg

Ginger-Soy Dressing

Low Cholesterol

Makes 1½ cups

¾ cup V8 vegetable juice
⅓ cup vegetable oil
2 tablespoons soy sauce
2 tablespoons red wine vinegar
1 tablespoon sugar
1 tablespoon grated fresh ginger
1 tablespoon dry sherry

In covered jar, combine all ingredients. Shake until well blended. Cover; refrigerate until serving time, at least 2 hours. Shake again before using. Serve over salad greens or pasta salads.

Nutrients per serving (1 tablespoon):

Calories	32	Sodium	109 mg
Fat	3 g	Cholesterol	0 mg

Stuffed Italian Zucchini

Low Cholesterol

Makes 4 servings

2 (7-inch) zucchini, cut in half lengthwise
½ cup chopped green pepper
½ cup chopped tomato
¼ cup chopped onion
½ teaspoon dried basil leaves, crushed
1 tablespoon PARKAY® Margarine
½ cup LIGHT N' LIVELY® Cottage Cheese
1 tablespoon KRAFT® 100% Grated Parmesan Cheese

Preheat oven to 350°. Trim ends of zucchini. Scoop out centers, leaving ¼-inch shell. Chop zucchini removed from centers. Sauté zucchini, peppers, tomatoes, onion and basil in margarine. Stir in cottage cheese. Spoon into shells; place in 9-inch square pan. Sprinkle with parmesan cheese. Bake 15 minutes.

Microwave Directions: Omit margarine. Prepare shells as directed. Microwave zucchini, peppers, tomatoes, onion and basil in microwave-safe 1½-quart bowl on High 2 to 4 minutes or until tender. Stir in cottage cheese. Spoon into shells; place in microwave-safe baking dish. Sprinkle with parmesan cheese. Microwave on High 2 to 3 minutes or until thoroughly heated.

Nutrients per serving:			
Calories	80	Sodium	140 mg
Fat	4 g	Cholesterol	5 mg

Almond Ratatouille

Quick & Easy

Makes 4 servings

¾ pound small new potatoes
2 tomatoes, chopped
1 medium eggplant, cubed (about 4 cups)
2 medium zucchini, sliced (about 2 cups)
1 red bell pepper, sliced
1 onion, thinly sliced
½ cup vegetable cocktail juice
2 tablespoons *each* chopped, fresh cilantro and lime juice
2 tablespoons Balsamic or red wine vinegar
1 tablespoon chopped fresh basil
2 cloves garlic, minced
1½ teaspoons chopped fresh dill°
⅓ cup blanched slivered almonds, toasted

Cut potatoes into bite-sized pieces. Place in 8×12-inch microwave-safe dish. Cover; microwave on High Power (100%) 2 minutes. Stir in remaining ingredients except almonds. Cover; microwave on High Power 15 minutes, stirring every 5 minutes until vegetables are tender-crisp and potatoes are cooked through. Remove from oven, stir in almonds and chill thoroughly before serving.

°Or use 1 teaspoon dried basil and ½ teaspoon dried dill.

Note: Hot Almond Ratatouille makes a wonderful topping for baked potatoes or broiled fish.

Nutrients per serving:			
Calories	145	Sodium	86 mg
Fat	4 g	Cholesterol	0 mg

Favorite recipe from **Almond Board of California.**

Ham Tortellini Salad

Quick & Easy

Makes 6 servings

1 (7- to 8-ounce) package cheese filled spinach tortellini
3 cups (12 ounces) ARMOUR® Lower Salt Ham, cut into ¾-inch cubes
½ cup sliced green onions
10 cherry tomatoes, cut in half
1 cup bottled low sodium, creamy buttermilk or reduced calorie zesty Italian salad dressing
   Leaf lettuce or butterhead lettuce, washed and drained
¼ cup finely chopped red pepper

Cook tortellini according to package directions omitting salt; drain and run under cold water to cool. Combine all ingredients *except* leaf lettuce and red pepper in large bowl. Toss until well blended. Serve on lettuce-lined salad plates. Sprinkle with red pepper. Serve immediately.

Nutrients per serving:			
Calories	165	Sodium	545 mg
Fat	4 g	Cholesterol	39 mg

Ham Tortellini Salad

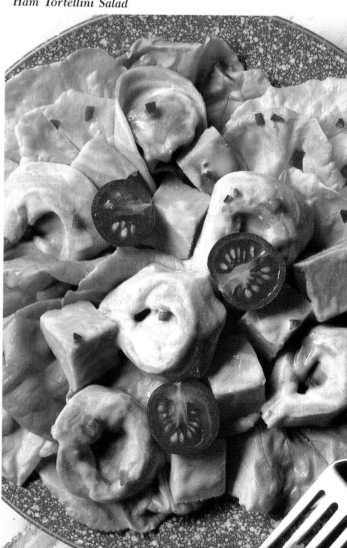

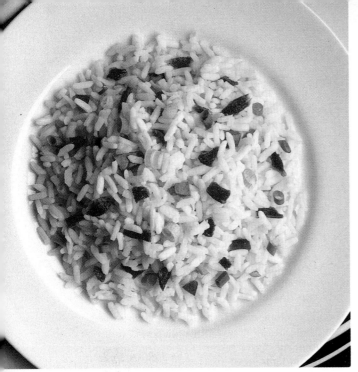

Bacon Pilaf

Bacon Pilaf

Low Cholesterol

Makes 4 to 6 servings

2 tablespoons unsalted margarine or butter
2 medium tomatoes, coarsely chopped
¼ cup sliced green onions
8 slices ARMOUR® Lower Salt Bacon, cooked crisp and crumbled
1 cup uncooked rice
1 teaspoon no salt added chicken flavor instant-bouillon

Melt margarine in large skillet or saucepan over medium heat. Add tomatoes and green onions; sauté for 2 minutes. Stir in 2 cups water and remaining ingredients. Heat to boiling; reduce heat and cover. Simmer about 20 to 25 minutes, or until liquid is absorbed. Fluff rice with fork before serving. Garnish with parsley, if desired.

Microwave Directions: Place margarine, tomatoes and green onions in large microwave-safe casserole dish. Cook, covered, on High power (100%) for 5 minutes. Add 2 cups water and remaining ingredients; cover. Cook on High power for 5 minutes. Reduce power to Medium-High (70%); cook about 10 to 12 minutes, or until liquid is absorbed. Let stand, covered, 5 minutes. Fluff rice with fork before serving. Garnish as above.

Nutrients per serving:			
Calories	197	Sodium	175 mg
Fat	8 g	Cholesterol	8 mg

Cashew-Shrimp Salad

Quick & Easy

Makes 4 cups or 4 servings

¾ cup V8 vegetable juice
1 tablespoon soy sauce
1 teaspoon vegetable oil
½ teaspoon grated lemon peel
½ teaspoon grated fresh ginger
¾ pound medium shrimp, cooked, shelled and deveined
1½ cups cucumber slices, cut in half
1 large carrot, cut into matchstick-thin strips (1¼ cups)
3 green onions, sliced (½ cup)
¼ cup coarsely chopped dry roasted unsalted cashews (1 ounce)
Lettuce leaves

1. In medium bowl, combine V8 juice, soy sauce, oil, lemon peel and ginger.

2. Add shrimp, cucumbers, carrot and green onions; toss to coat well. Cover; refrigerate until serving time, at least 2 hours.

3. Before serving, add cashews; toss to coat well. To serve: On 4 lettuce-lined salad plates, arrange shrimp mixture.

Nutrients per serving:			
Calories	162	Sodium	526 mg
Fat	5 g	Cholesterol	106 mg

Corn Olé

Low Sodium

Makes 6 servings

2 tablespoons butter or margarine
3 cups chopped fresh tomatoes
2 cups fresh corn, cut off the cob (about 4 ears)
2 cups (about ¾ pound) summer squash slices, halved
⅓ cup chopped onion
¼ teaspoon pepper

Melt butter in large skillet. Add remaining ingredients; cover. Cook 10 to 15 minutes or until squash is tender, stirring occasionally.

Nutrients per serving:			
Calories	127	Sodium	58 mg
Fat	5 g	Cholesterol	10 mg

Favorite recipe from United Fresh Fruit and Vegetable Association.

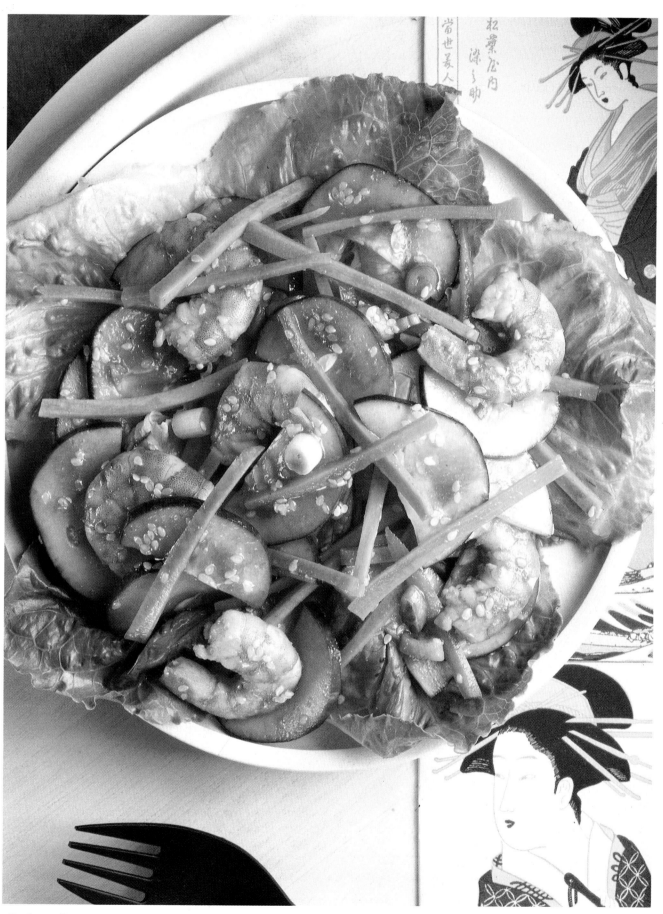

Cashew-Shrimp Salad

Colorful Cauliflower Bake

Low Cholesterol

Makes 6 servings

1 cup KELLOGG'S® ALL-BRAN® cereal
2 tablespoons margarine, melted
¼ teaspoon garlic salt
¼ cup flour
½ teaspoon salt
⅛ teaspoon white pepper
1⅓ cups skim milk
1 chicken bouillon cube
1 package (16 oz.) frozen, cut cauliflower, thawed, well-drained
½ cup sliced green onions
2 tablespoons drained, chopped pimento

1. Combine KELLOGG'S® ALL-BRAN® cereal, margarine and garlic salt; set aside.

2. In 3-quart saucepan, combine flour, salt and pepper. Gradually add milk, mixing until smooth, using a wire whip if necessary. Add bouillon cube. Cook, stirring constantly, over medium heat until bubbly and thickened. Remove from heat.

3. Add cauliflower, onions and pimento, mixing until combined. Spread evenly in 1½-quart serving dish. Sprinkle with cereal mixture.

4. Bake at 350° about 20 minutes or until thoroughly heated and sauce is bubbly.

Note: 3½ cups fresh cauliflower flowerets, cooked crisp-tender, may be substituted for frozen cauliflower.

Nutrients per serving:			
Calories	120	Sodium	508 mg
Fat	4 g	Cholesterol	1 mg

Caribbean Yam Bake

Low Sodium

Makes 6 servings

3 cups cooked, mashed yams (2 pounds)
2 eggs
½ cup brown sugar, packed
¼ cup margarine, melted
2 tablespoons dark rum (optional)
½ teaspoon ground nutmeg
  Zest and juice from 1 lime
2 DOLE® Bananas, peeled, diced

In large bowl, combine mashed yams with eggs, brown sugar, margarine, rum (if used), nutmeg, lime zest and juice until thoroughly mixed. Fold in diced bananas. Turn into shallow greased 5-cup baking dish. Bake in 375°F oven 40 minutes.

Nutrients per serving:			
Calories	290	Sodium	125 mg
Fat	10 g	Cholesterol	91 mg

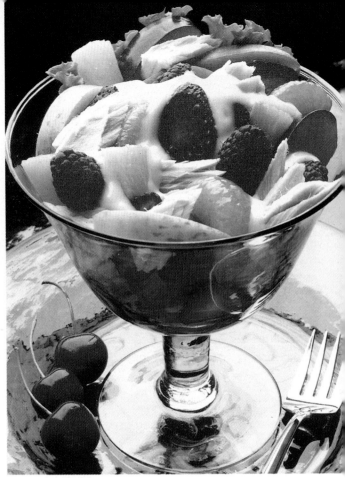

Tuna & Fresh Fruit Salad

Tuna & Fresh Fruit Salad

Quick & Easy

Makes 4 servings

  Lettuce leaves (optional)
1 can (12½ ounces) STARKIST® Tuna, drained and broken into chunks
4 cups slices or wedges fresh fruit°
¼ cup silvered almonds (optional)

Fruit Dressing
1 container (8 ounces) lemon, mandarin orange or vanilla low-fat yogurt
2 tablespoons orange juice
¼ teaspoon ground cinnamon

Line a large platter or 4 individual plates with lettuce leaves, if desired. Arrange tuna and desired fruit in a decorative design over lettuce. Sprinkle almonds over salad if desired.

For Fruit Dressing: In a small bowl stir together yogurt, orange juice and cinnamon until well blended. Serve dressing with salad.

°Suggested fresh fruit: Apples, bananas, berries, citrus fruit, kiwifruit, melon, papaya, peaches or pears.

Nutrients per serving (including ¼ cup dressing):			
Calories	233	Sodium	434 mg
Fat	1 g	Cholesterol	39 mg

Baked Tomatoes Florentine

Makes 4 servings

1 cup sliced fresh mushrooms (optional)
1 tablespoon finely chopped onion
¼ cup water
1 cup BORDEN® Lite-line® skim milk
3 tablespoons flour
2 teaspoons WYLER'S® Chicken-Flavor Instant
    Bouillon
6 slices BORDEN® Lite-line® Process Cheese
    Product, any flavor, cut into small pieces°
2 cups cubed cooked chicken (white meat)
1 (10-ounce) package frozen chopped spinach or
    broccoli, thawed and well drained
4 large tomatoes, tops cut off and insides scooped
    out

Preheat oven to 350°. In small saucepan, cook mushrooms, if desired, and onion in water until tender; drain. In small saucepan, combine milk, flour and bouillon; over low heat, cook and stir until thickened. Add Lite-line® pieces; cook and stir until melted. In medium bowl, combine mushroom mixture, chicken, spinach and ¾ *cup* sauce; stuff tomatoes. Arrange in baking dish; cover and bake 15 to 20 minutes or until hot. Over low heat, heat remaining sauce with 1 to 2 tablespoons water. Spoon over tomatoes before serving. Garnish as desired. Refrigerate leftovers.

°"½ the calories" 8% milkfat version

Nutrients per serving:			
Calories	290	Sodium	1053 mg
Fat	6 g	Cholesterol	71 mg

Baked Tomatoes Florentine

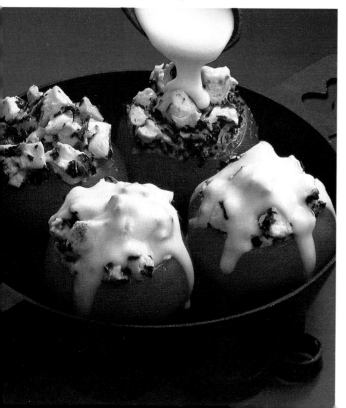

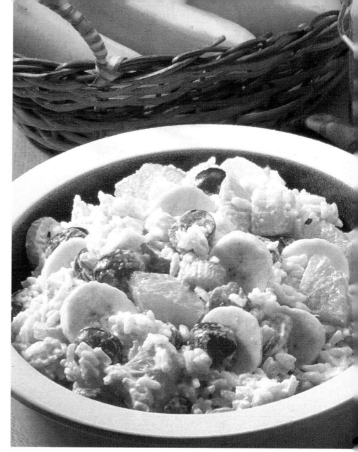

Curried Fruit and Rice Salad

Curried Fruit and Rice Salad

Makes 6 servings

2 cups cooked rice, chilled
1 orange, sliced and quartered
1 cup red seedless grapes, halved
⅓ cup mayonnaise
⅓ cup vanilla yogurt
½ teaspoon curry powder, or to taste
    Zest and juice from 1 lime
1 DOLE® Banana, peeled, sliced

Combine rice, orange and grapes. Combine mayonnaise, yogurt, curry, lime zest and juice; stir dressing into salad. Fold in banana just before serving.

Nutrients per serving:			
Calories	189	Sodium	76 mg
Fat	10 g	Cholesterol	9 mg

Springtime Vegetable Slaw

Makes 10 servings

  1 pound shredded DOLE® Cabbage
  1 cup grated DOLE® Carrots
  ½ cup DOLE® Broccoli flowerets, chopped
  ½ cup halved cherry tomatoes
  ½ cup sliced DOLE® Celery
  ½ cup peeled, seeded, diced DOLE® Cucumber
  1 cup chopped DOLE® Parsley
  ⅓ cup olive oil
  2 tablespoons vinegar
  1 tablespoon Dijon mustard
  1 teaspoon garlic salt

Combine cabbage, carrots, broccoli, tomatoes, celery and cucumber in salad bowl. Whisk together remaining ingredients for dressing. Toss salad with dressing.

Nutrients per serving:

Calories	87	Sodium	147 mg
Fat	7 g	Cholesterol	0 mg

Springtime Vegetable Slaw

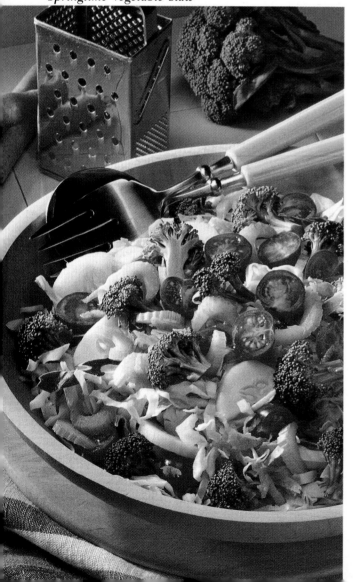

Lemony Apple-Bran Salad

Makes 6 servings

  ½ cup plain low-fat yogurt
  1 tablespoon chopped parsley
  1 teaspoon sugar
  1 teaspoon lemon juice
  ½ teaspoon salt
  2 cups chopped, cored red apples
  ½ cup thinly sliced celery
  ½ cup halved, green grapes *or* ¼ cup raisins
  ½ cup KELLOGG'S® All-Bran® cereal

1. In medium-size bowl, combine yogurt, parsley, sugar, lemon juice and salt. Stir in apples, celery and grapes or raisins. Cover and refrigerate until ready to serve.

2. Just before serving, stir in KELLOGG'S® All-Bran® cereal. Serve on lettuce, if desired.

Nutrients per serving:

Calories	60	Sodium	260 mg
Fat	1 g	Cholesterol	1 mg

Crispened New Potatoes

Makes 4 servings

1½ lbs. very small, scrubbed new potatoes
    (about 12)
  ½ cup QUAKER® Oat Bran hot cereal, uncooked
  2 tablespoons grated parmesan cheese
  1 tablespoon snipped fresh parsley *or* 1 teaspoon
    dried parsley flakes
  ½ teaspoon snipped fresh dill *or* ½ teaspoon dried
    dill weed
  ½ teaspoon paprika
  ¼ cup skim milk
  1 egg white, slightly beaten
  1 tablespoon margarine, melted

Heat oven to 400°F. Lightly spray 11×7-inch dish with vegetable oil cooking spray or oil lightly. Cook whole potatoes in boiling water 15 minutes. Drain; rinse in cold water.

In shallow dish, combine oat bran, cheese, parsley, dill and paprika. In another shallow dish, combine milk and egg white. Coat each potato in oat bran mixture; shake off excess. Dip into egg mixture, then coat again with oat bran mixture. Place into prepared dish; drizzle with margarine. Cover; bake 10 minutes. Uncover; bake an additional 10 minutes or until potatoes are tender.

Nutrients per serving:

Calories	230	Sodium	110 mg
Fat	5 g	Cholesterol	0 mg

Creamy Fruit Mold

Low Cholesterol

Makes 7 servings

1 package (0.3 ounces) sugar free lime flavor
   gelatin
1 cup boiling water
1 cup PET® Light Evaporated Skimmed Milk
2 cups fresh fruit, cut-up°

Dissolve gelatin in boiling water. Cool slightly to
prevent milk from curdling. Stir in evaporated
skimmed milk. Chill until the consistency of unbeaten
egg whites. Stir in fruit. Pour into an 8-inch square
pan or a 5-cup mold. Chill until firm. Garnish with
additional fruit.

°*Suggested fresh fruit: Apples, bing cherries, oranges,
peaches or strawberries.*

Nutrients per serving:

Calories	51	Sodium	77 mg
Fat	0 g	Cholesterol	1 mg

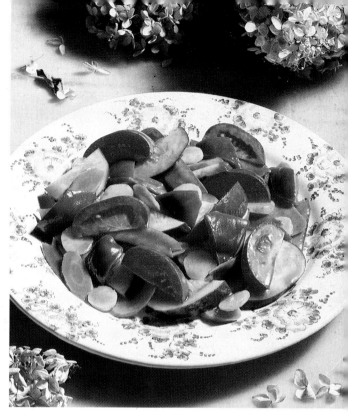

Sweet 'n Sour Stir-Fry

California Fruit Salad Rosé

Low Sodium

Makes 8 servings

1 envelope KNOX® Unflavored Gelatine
¾ cup cold water
1¼ cups rosé wine
2 tablespoons sugar
   Fresh fruit°

In medium saucepan, sprinkle unflavored gelatine
over cold water; let stand 1 minute. Stir over low heat
until gelatine is completely dissolved, about 5
minutes. Stir in wine and sugar until sugar is
dissolved. Chill, stirring occasionally, until mixture is
consistency of unbeaten egg whites, about 60 minutes.
Fold in suggested fresh fruit. Pour into wine glasses
or 4-cup mold; chill until firm, about 3 hours. To
serve, unmold onto platter.

°*Suggested fresh fruit: Use any combination of the
following to equal 2 cups—sliced bananas,
blueberries, grapes, cut-up melon, peaches, raspberries
or strawberries.*

Nutrients per serving:

Calories	62	Sodium	4 mg
Fat	0 g	Cholesterol	0 mg

Sweet 'n Sour Stir-Fry

Low Cholesterol

Makes 6 servings

2 tablespoons oil
1 cup thinly sliced carrots
1 cup snow peas (about 4 ounces)
1 small green bell pepper, cut into chunks
1 cup sliced water chestnuts
1 medium tomato, cut into wedges
½ cup sliced cucumber, halved
¾ cup WISH-BONE® Lite Sweet 'n Sour Spicy
   French Dressing
2 tablespoons brown sugar
2 teaspoons soy sauce

In medium skillet, heat oil and cook carrots, snow
peas and green bell pepper over medium heat,
stirring frequently, 5 minutes or until crisp-tender.
Add water chestnuts, tomato, cucumber and sweet 'n
sour spicy French dressing blended with brown sugar
and soy sauce. Simmer, covered, 5 minutes or until
vegetables are tender. Top, if desired, with sesame
seeds.

Nutrients per serving:

Calories	137	Sodium	348 mg
Fat	5 g	Cholesterol	0 mg

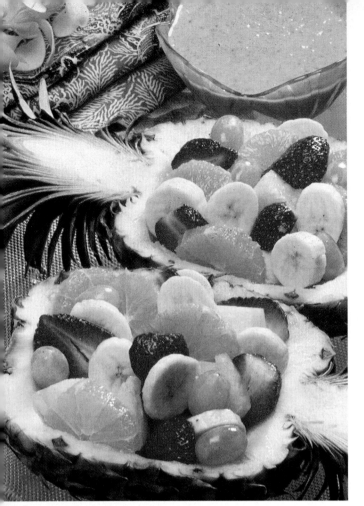

Summer Fruit Salad

Summer Fruit Salad

Low Sodium

Makes 6 servings

1 DOLE® Fresh Pineapple
2 DOLE® Oranges, peeled, sliced
2 DOLE® Bananas, peeled, sliced
1 cup halved DOLE® Strawberries
1 cup seedless green DOLE® Grapes
   Strawberry-Banana Yogurt Dressing (recipe
   follows)
   Orange-Banana Yogurt Dressing (recipe follows)

Cut pineapple in half lengthwise through crown. Remove fruit with curved knife, leaving shells intact. Trim off core and cut fruit into chunks. In large bowl, combine pineapple, oranges, bananas, strawberries and grapes. Spoon into pineapple shells. Serve with your choice of dressing.

Strawberry-Banana Yogurt Dressing

6 DOLE® Strawberries, halved
1 ripe DOLE® Banana, peeled
1 carton (8 ounces) vanilla yogurt
1 tablespoon brown sugar or honey

In blender or food processor, combine all ingredients and blend until smooth.

Orange-Banana Yogurt Dressing

1 DOLE® Orange
1 ripe DOLE® Banana, peeled
1 carton (8 ounces) vanilla yogurt
1 tablespoon brown sugar or honey

Grate peel from ½ orange. Juice orange (⅓ cup). In blender or food processor, combine orange peel and juice with remaining ingredients. Blend until smooth.

Nutrients per serving (with 1 tablespoon Strawberry-Banana Dressing):

Calories	143	Sodium	15 mg
Fat	2 g	Cholesterol	4 mg

Citrus Cheese Salad

Quick & Easy

Makes 1 serving

½ cup BORDEN® Lite-line® lowfat cottage cheese
1 slice BORDEN® Lite-line® Process Cheese
   Product, any flavor, cut into small pieces°
2 tablespoons chopped cucumber
½ fresh grapefruit, pared and sectioned
   Lettuce leaf

In small bowl, combine cottage cheese, Lite-line® pieces and cucumber. On salad plate, arrange grapefruit on lettuce. Top with cheese mixture. Refrigerate leftovers.

°"½ the calories" 8% milkfat version

Nutrients per serving:

Calories	200	Sodium	714 mg
Fat	3 g	Cholesterol	15 mg

Citrus Cheese Salad

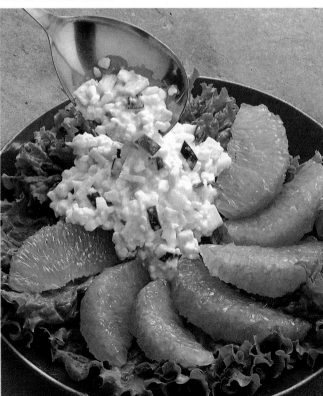

Family Baked Bean Dinner

Makes 6 servings

1 can (20 ounces) DOLE® Pineapple Chunks
½ green bell pepper, cut in strips
½ cup chopped onion
⅓ cup brown sugar, packed
1 teaspoon dry mustard
2 cans (16 ounces *each*) baked beans

Drain pineapple. Add green pepper and onion to 12×8-inch microwave dish. Cover, microwave on HIGH 3 minutes. In a mixing bowl, combine brown sugar and mustard; stir in beans and pineapple. Add to green pepper mixture. Stir to combine. Microwave, uncovered, on HIGH 8 to 10 minutes, stirring after 4 minutes. Serve with Polish sausage or hot dogs if desired.

Nutrients per serving:

Calories	273	Sodium	678 mg
Fat	1 g	Cholesterol	0 mg

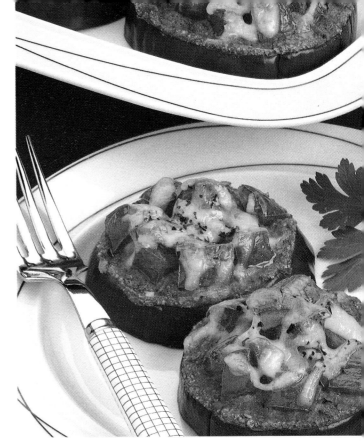

Eggplant Italiano

Spinach Salad with Raspberry Dressing

Makes 2 servings

½ cup plain nonfat yogurt
¼ cup fresh or frozen red raspberries, thawed if frozen
1 tablespoon skim milk
1½ teaspoons chopped fresh mint *or* ½ teaspoon dried mint, crushed
4 to 6 cups fresh spinach, washed, drained and trimmed
2 large fresh mushrooms, sliced
1 tablespoon sesame seeds, toasted
4 to 6 red onion rings
6 slices ARMOUR® Lower Salt Bacon, cooked crisp and crumbled

Carefully combine yogurt, raspberries, milk and mint in small bowl; set aside. Combine spinach, mushrooms and sesame seeds in medium bowl; mix well. Arrange spinach mixture evenly on 2 individual salad plates; top with red onion rings. Drizzle yogurt dressing over salads; sprinkle with bacon. Garnish with fresh raspberries and mint sprig, if desired.

Nutrients per serving:

Calories	200	Sodium	556 mg
Fat	10 g	Cholesterol	19 mg

Eggplant Italiano

Makes 4 servings

1 eggplant (1 lb.), peeled if desired
1 can (6 oz.) low sodium cocktail vegetable juice (¾ cup)
½ cup QUAKER® Oat Bran hot cereal, uncooked
2 garlic cloves, minced
1 teaspoon basil leaves, crushed
½ teaspoon oregano
2 medium tomatoes, chopped
1¼ cups (5 oz.) shredded part skim mozzarella cheese

Heat oven to 350°. Line cookie sheet or 15×10-inch baking pan with foil. Lightly spray with vegetable oil cooking spray or oil lightly. Cut eggplant into ½-inch-thick slices; place in single layer on prepared pan. Combine vegetable juice, oat bran, garlic, basil and oregano. Spread evenly over eggplant; top with tomatoes. Sprinkle with mozzarella cheese. Bake 35 to 40 minutes or until eggplant is tender and cheese is melted. Sprinkle with additional basil or oregano, if desired.

Nutrients per serving:

Calories	190	Sodium	190 mg
Fat	7 g	Cholesterol	20 mg

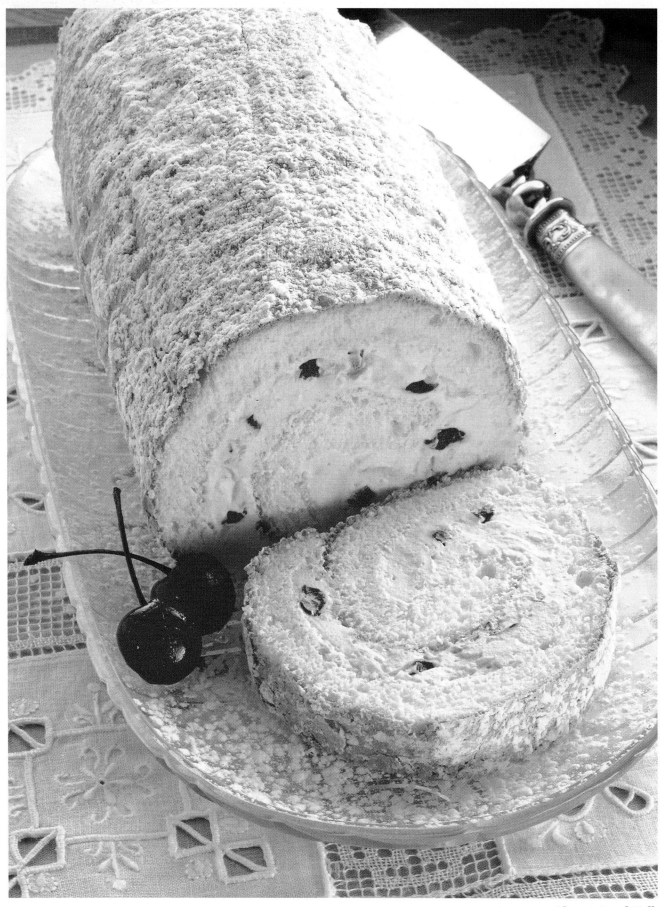

Cherry Angel Rolls

Desserts

Cherry Angel Rolls

> **Low Cholesterol**

Makes 16 servings

1 package DUNCAN HINES® Angel Food Cake Mix
1 cup chopped maraschino cherries, drained
½ cup flaked coconut
1 teaspoon maraschino cherry juice
1 container (8 ounces) frozen whipped topping, thawed
Confectioners' sugar

1. Preheat oven to 350°F. Line two 15½×10½×1-inch jelly roll pans with aluminum foil.

2. Prepare cake following package directions. Divide batter into lined pans. Spread evenly. Cut through batter with knife or spatula to remove large air bubbles. Bake at 350°F for 15 minutes or until set. Immediately invert cakes onto towels covered with confectioners' sugar. Remove foil carefully. Immediately roll up each cake with towel jelly roll fashion. Cool completely.

3. Fold cherries, coconut and cherry juice into whipped topping. Unroll cakes. Spread half of filling over each cake to edges. Reroll and place seam-side down on serving plate. Dust with confectioners' sugar. Refrigerate until ready to serve.

Tip: Use clean, lint-free dishtowels to roll up cakes.

Nutrients per serving:

Calories	211	Sodium	113 mg
Fat	6 g	Cholesterol	0 mg

Very Berry Sorbet

> **Low Cholesterol**

Makes 8 servings

1 envelope KNOX® Unflavored Gelatine
½ cup sugar
1½ cups water
2 cups puréed strawberries or raspberries (about 1½ pints)°
½ cup crème de cassis (black currant) liqueur or cranberry juice cocktail
2 tablespoons lemon juice

In medium saucepan, mix unflavored gelatine with sugar; blend in water. Let stand 1 minute. Stir over low heat until gelatine is completely dissolved, about 5 minutes. Let cool to room temperature; stir in remaining ingredients. Pour into 9-inch square baking pan; freeze 3 hours or until firm.

With electric mixer or food processor, beat mixture until smooth. Return to pan; freeze 2 hours or until firm. To serve, let stand at room temperature 15 minutes or until slightly softened. Spoon into dessert dishes or stemmed glassware. Garnish, if desired, with fresh fruit.

°Substitution: Use 1 package (10 ounces) frozen strawberries or raspberries, partially thawed and puréed.

Nutrients per serving:

Calories	111	Sodium	2 mg
Fat	0 g	Cholesterol	0 mg

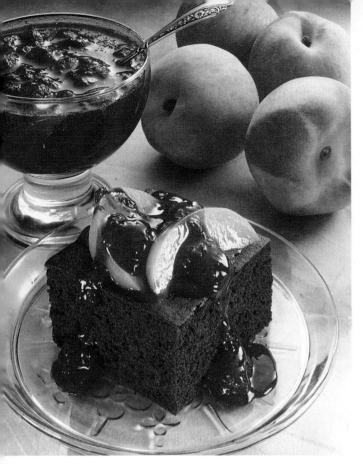

Fudge Cake with Melba Topping

Fudge Cake with Melba Topping

Low Cholesterol

Makes 20 servings

Cake
   1 package DUNCAN HINES® Moist Deluxe
      Dark Dutch Fudge Cake Mix
   Egg substitute product equal to 3 eggs
1¼ cups water
½ cup PURITAN® Oil

Raspberry Sauce
   1 package (12 ounces) frozen dry pack
      raspberries, thawed, drained and juice
      reserved
½ cup sugar
2 teaspoons cornstarch
½ teaspoon grated lemon peel

   1 can (29 ounces) sliced peaches in lite syrup,
      drained

1. Preheat oven to 350°F. Grease and flour 13×9×2-inch pan.

2. For cake: Combine cake mix, egg substitute, water and oil in large bowl. Beat at medium speed with electric mixer for 2 minutes. Pour into pan. Bake at 350°F for 35 to 40 minutes or until toothpick inserted in center comes out clean. Cool completely.

3. For sauce: Combine reserved raspberry juice, sugar, cornstarch and lemon peel in medium saucepan. Bring to a boil. Reduce heat and cook until thickened, stirring constantly. Stir in reserved raspberries. Cool.

4. Cut cake into serving squares. Place several peach slices on top of cake square. Spoon raspberry sauce over peaches and cake. Serve immediately.

Tip: To separate juice from raspberries in one step, allow berries to thaw at room temperature in a strainer placed over a bowl.

Nutrients per serving:			
Calories	199	Sodium	231 mg
Fat	9 g	Cholesterol	0 mg

Carrot Raisin Cake

Low Sodium

Makes 16 servings

Cake
  ½ cup CRISCO® Shortening
1½ cups sugar
  2 eggs
  1 egg white
  ¼ cup skim milk
2⅓ cups all-purpose flour
  2 teaspoons baking soda
  1 teaspoon cinnamon
  ½ teaspoon baking powder
  ½ teaspoon salt (optional)
  2 cups finely shredded carrots (about 4 medium)
⅔ cup raisins

Topping°
  1 teaspoon powdered sugar

1. Heat oven 350°F. Grease and flour 12-cup Bundt® pan.

2. For cake: Cream CRISCO®, sugar, eggs and egg white at medium speed of electric mixer until light and fluffy. Add milk, flour, baking soda, cinnamon, baking powder and salt (if used). Beat at low speed until blended, scraping bowl constantly. Beat at medium speed for 2 minutes, scraping bowl occasionally. Stir in carrots and raisins. Turn into pan. Spread evenly.

3. Bake at 350°F for 50 to 55 minutes or until wooden pick inserted in center comes out clean. Cool in pan for 5 minutes. Invert on wire rack. Cool completely.

4. For topping: Sprinkle cake with powdered sugar.

°Optional yogurt topping: Combine 1 cup plain nonfat or lowfat yogurt with 3 tablespoons brown sugar and ½ teaspoon vanilla. Spoon over cake slices.

Nutrients per serving (without topping):			
Calories	230	Sodium	135 mg
Fat	7 g	Cholesterol	35 mg

Cinnamon Fruit Tart with Sour Cream Filling

Low Cholesterol

Makes 12 servings

- 1 envelope KNOX® Unflavored Gelatine
- ¼ cup cold water
- 1 cup (8 ounces) creamed cottage cheese
- ¾ cup pineapple juice
- ½ cup sour cream
- ½ cup milk
- ¼ cup sugar
- 1 teaspoon lemon juice
- Cinnamon Graham Cracker Crust (recipe follows)
- Suggested fresh fruit°
- 2 tablespoons orange or apricot marmalade, melted

In small saucepan, sprinkle unflavored gelatine over cold water; let stand 1 minute. Stir over low heat until gelatine is completely dissolved, about 3 minutes.

In blender or food processor, process cottage cheese, pineapple juice, sour cream, milk, sugar and lemon juice until blended. While processing, through feed cap, gradually add gelatine mixture and process until blended. Pour into Cinnamon Graham Cracker Crust; chill until firm, about 3 hours. To serve: Top with suggested fresh fruit, then brush with marmalade.

Cinnamon Graham Cracker Crust: In small bowl, combine 2 cups graham cracker crumbs, 1 tablespoon sugar, ½ teaspoon ground cinnamon and ¼ cup melted butter. Press into 10-inch tart pan. Bake at 375°, 8 minutes; cool.

°*Suggested fresh fruit: Use any combination of the following to equal 2 cups — blueberries, kiwi, oranges, raspberries or sliced strawberries.*

Nutrients per serving:			
Calories	212	Sodium	248 mg
Fat	8 g	Cholesterol	19 mg

Cinnamon Fruit Tart with Sour Cream Filling

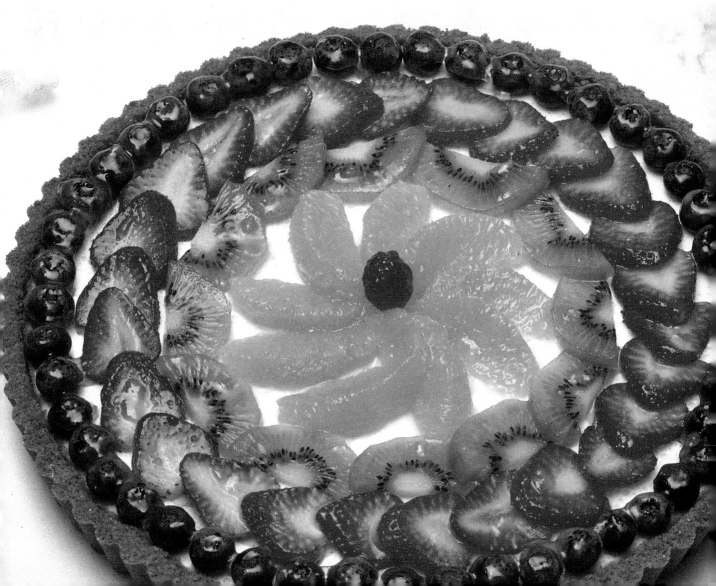

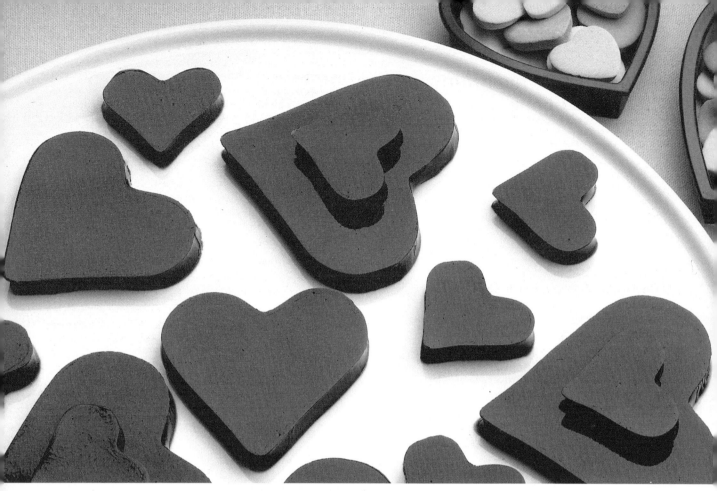

Jell-O® Sugar Free Jigglers Gelatin Snacks

Jell-O® Sugar Free Jigglers Gelatin Snacks

Low Sodium

Makes about 8 dozen cubes

2½ cups boiling water
  4 packages (4-serving size each) or 2 packages
    (8-serving size each) JELL-O® Brand Sugar
      Free Gelatin, any flavor

ADD boiling water to gelatin. Dissolve completely.
Pour into 13×9-inch pan. Chill until firm, about 3
hours.

DIP pan in warm water about 15 seconds for easy
removal. Cut gelatin into 1-inch squares. (Or use
cookie cutters to cut decorative shapes; cut remaining
gelatin into cubes.)

*Notes: For thicker JELL-O® Sugar Free Jigglers, use
8- or 9-inch square pan.*

*To use ice cube trays or JELL-O® Jiggler molds, pour
gelatin mixture into 2 or 3 ice cube trays. Chill until
firm, about 2 hours. To remove, dip trays in warm
water about 15 seconds. Moisten tips of fingers and
gently pull from edges.*

Nutrients per serving:

Calories	2	Sodium	10 mg
Fat	0 g	Cholesterol	0 mg

Spice Cookies

Low Cholesterol

Makes 2½ dozen cookies

1½ cups all-purpose flour
  ½ teaspoon baking soda
  ¼ teaspoon cinnamon
  ¼ teaspoon nutmeg
  ½ cup margarine, softened
  1 cup firmly packed brown sugar
  2 egg whites
  2 cups KELLOGG'S® COMMON SENSE™ Oat
    Bran cereal, any variety

1. Stir together flour, soda and spices; set aside.

2. In large bowl, beat together margarine, sugar and
egg whites. Add flour mixture and beat until
combined. Mix in KELLOGG'S® COMMON
SENSE™ Oat Bran cereal. Drop by level measuring-
tablespoon onto ungreased baking sheets.

3. Bake in 375°F oven about 9 minutes or until lightly
browned.

Nutrients per serving (2 cookies):

Calories	190	Sodium	176 mg
Fat	6 g	Cholesterol	0 mg

Creamy Lemon Cheesecake

Low Cholesterol

Makes 8 servings

Crust
 1 cup graham cracker crumbs
 ¼ cup sugar
 3 tablespoons PURITAN® Oil

Filling
 2 cups low-fat (1%) cottage cheese
 3 ounces neufchatel cheese
 2 egg whites
 ½ cup sugar
 3 tablespoons fresh lemon juice
 1 teaspoon freshly grated lemon peel
 1 teaspoon vanilla

1. Heat oven to 350°F.

2. For crust: Combine graham cracker crumbs, sugar and PURITAN® Oil in 9-inch pie plate. Mix well with fork. Press firmly against bottom and halfway up sides of pie plate.

3. For filling: Blend cheeses in food processor or blender°, until completely smooth. Add remaining ingredients. Blend well. Pour mixture into crust.

4. Bake at 350°F for 30 minutes. Turn oven off and allow cheesecake to remain in oven for 5 minutes. Remove from oven. Cool to room temperature, then chill.

5. Cut in wedges. Garnish with fresh fruit, if desired.

°If blender is used, place egg whites, sugar, lemon juice, lemon peel and vanilla in blender container before adding neufchatel and cottage cheese. Blend until completely smooth, stopping blender and scraping as necessary.

Microwave Directions:
1. Prepare crumb mixture as above. Spoon 2 to 3 tablespoons crumb mixture into 8 small custard cups. Press firmly against bottoms of cups. Prepare filling as above. Pour about ⅓ cup filling into each cup.

2. Arrange cups in circle on large microwave-safe platter or directly on floor of microwave oven. Microwave on Medium 9 to 10 minutes, or until filling begins to set around edges, turning platter or rearranging cups after each 3 minutes.

3. Let stand on countertop or board 10 minutes. Chill 1 hour or longer.

Nutrients per serving:			
Calories	240	Sodium	330 mg
Fat	9 g	Cholesterol	10 mg

Strawberries 'n Cream Fool

Low Cholesterol

Makes 8 servings

 1 envelope KNOX® Unflavored Gelatine
 ¼ cup cold water
 1 package (10 ounces) frozen strawberries in light syrup, thawed
 ¼ cup frozen orange juice concentrate, partially thawed and undiluted
 ¼ cup sugar
 1 teaspoon finely chopped crystallized ginger (optional)
 1 container (8 ounces) frozen whipped topping, thawed

In medium saucepan, sprinkle unflavored gelatine over cold water; let stand 1 minute. Stir over low heat until gelatine is completely dissolved, about 3 minutes.

In blender or food processor, process strawberries, orange juice concentrate, sugar and ginger. While processing, through feed cap, gradually add gelatine mixture and process until blended. In large bowl, blend 1 cup strawberry mixture with whipped topping. Turn into serving bowl. Gently fold in remaining strawberry mixture, just until marbled; chill until set, about 2 hours. Serve, if desired, with angel food or pound cake.

Nutrients per serving:			
Calories	165	Sodium	9 mg
Fat	7 g	Cholesterol	0 mg

Lite Chocolate Sauce

Quick & Easy

Makes ¾ cup sauce

 2 tablespoons regular margarine
 ¼ cup plus 2 tablespoons sugar
 2 tablespoons HERSHEY'S® Cocoa
 2 tablespoons light corn syrup
 ¼ cup evaporated skim milk
 1 teaspoon vanilla

In small saucepan over low heat melt margarine. Remove from heat; stir in sugar, cocoa and corn syrup. Add evaporated skim milk. Cook over low heat, stirring constantly, just until mixture begins to boil and is smooth. Remove from heat; stir in vanilla. Cool slightly. Spoon 1 tablespoon warm sauce over ½ cup vanilla ice milk for each serving.

Nutrients per serving (1 tablespoon sauce):			
Calories	152	Sodium	86 mg
Fat	5 g	Cholesterol	9 mg

French Vanilla Fruit Delight

Low Cholesterol

Makes 16 servings

1 package DUNCAN HINES® Moist Deluxe
    French Vanilla Cake Mix
1 can (8¾ ounces) unpeeled apricot halves,
    drained
1 jar (12 ounces) apricot preserves

1. Preheat oven to 350°F. Grease and flour 10-inch tube pan. Prepare, bake and cool cake following package directions for no-cholesterol recipe.

2. Arrange apricots on top of cake. Heat apricot preserves until warm. Pour over apricot slices and cake. Refrigerate until ready to serve.

Tip: For delicious flavor variation, try substituting raspberry or strawberry preserves in place of apricot.

Nutrients per serving:			
Calories	258	Sodium	225 mg
Fat	7 g	Cholesterol	0 mg

Oatmeal Raisin Cookies

Low Cholesterol

Makes 4 dozen cookies

½ cup CRISCO® Shortening
1¼ cups firmly packed brown sugar
2 egg whites
⅓ cup skim milk
2 teaspoons vanilla
3 cups quick oats (not instant or old fashioned)
1 cup all-purpose flour
½ teaspoon salt (optional)
½ teaspoon baking soda
½ teaspoon cinnamon
1 cup raisins

1. Heat oven to 375°F. Grease baking sheet.

2. Combine CRISCO®, brown sugar, egg whites, milk and vanilla in large bowl. Beat at medium speed of electric mixer for 1½ minutes. Scrape sides of bowl frequently (batter may appear slightly curdled).

3. Combine oats, flour, salt (if used), baking soda and cinnamon in separate bowl. Beat into above mixture at low speed until blended. Stir in raisins.

4. Drop by slightly rounded measuring tablespoonfuls onto baking sheet.

5. Bake at 375°F for 8 or 9 minutes or until lightly browned. Cool on baking sheet for 2 minutes. Remove to wire rack.

Nutrients per serving (2 cookies):			
Calories	170	Sodium	25 mg
Fat	5 g	Cholesterol	0 mg

Refreshing Cocoa-Fruit Sherbet

Low Sodium

Makes 8 servings

1 medium-size ripe banana
1½ cups orange juice
1 cup half-and-half
½ cup sugar
¼ cup HERSHEY'S® Cocoa

Slice banana into blender container. Add orange juice; blend until smooth. Add remaining ingredients; blend well. Pour into 9-inch square pan or two ice cube trays; freeze until hard around edges. Spoon mixture into blender container or large mixer bowl; blend until smooth. Pour into 1-quart mold; freeze until firm. To serve, unmold onto chilled plate and slice.

Nutrients per serving:			
Calories	131	Sodium	14 mg
Fat	3 g	Cholesterol	11 mg

Peachy Snack Cake

Low Sodium

Makes 12 servings

2 tablespoons margarine, melted
¼ cup firmly packed brown sugar
3 cups KELLOGG'S® Raisin Bran cereal, divided
1 cup all-purpose flour
¼ teaspoon salt
1 teaspoon baking powder
1 teaspoon cinnamon
¼ teaspoon nutmeg
¼ cup margarine, softened
½ cup granulated sugar
2 eggs
1 can (16 oz.) sliced cling peaches, drained, cut
    into bite-size pieces

1. In small bowl, combine 2 tablespoons margarine, brown sugar and 1½ cups cereal; set aside.

2. Combine flour, salt, baking powder and spices; set aside.

3. In medium-size bowl, beat together ¼ cup margarine, granulated sugar and eggs until well combined. Stir in peaches. Add flour mixture and remaining 1½ cups cereal, stirring until combined. Spread evenly in greased 9-inch square baking pan. Sprinkle with prepared topping.

4. Bake in 350°F oven about 30 minutes or until cake tester comes out clean. Serve warm or cold.

Nutrients per serving:			
Calories	210	Sodium	243 mg
Fat	7 g	Cholesterol	46 mg

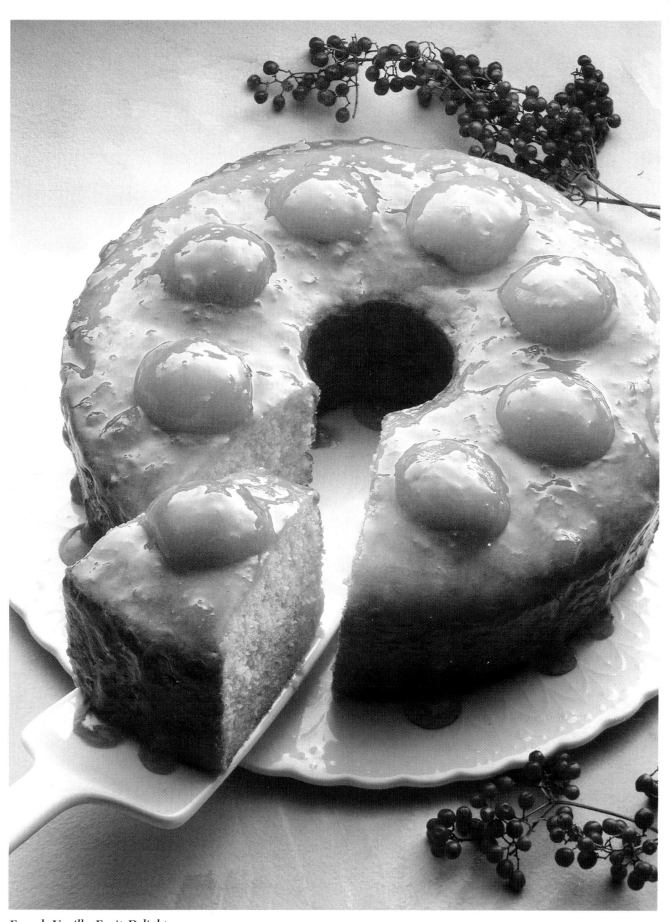

French Vanilla Fruit Delight

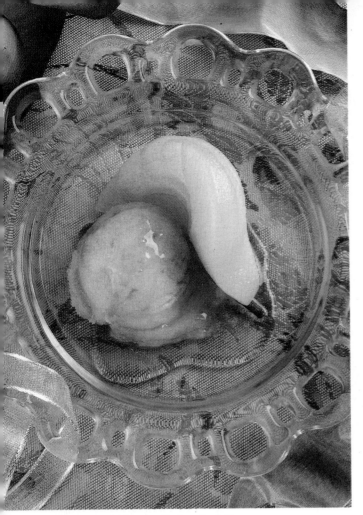

Zinfandel Sorbet with Poached Pears.

Zinfandel Sorbet with Poached Pears

Low Cholesterol

Makes 8 servings

Zinfandel Sorbet
  1 envelope KNOX® Unflavored Gelatine
  ½ cup cold water
  ⅓ cup sugar
  1¼ cups white Zinfandel wine
  1 can (5½ ounces) pear nectar

Poached Pears
  2 cups white Zinfandel wine
  ¾ cup sugar
  1 tablespoon lemon juice
  4 medium Anjou or Bartlett pears, peeled, halved, and cored

Zinfandel Sorbet: In medium saucepan, sprinkle unflavored gelatine over cold water; let stand 1 minute. Stir over low heat until gelatine is completely dissolved, about 3 minutes. Stir in sugar until dissolved, then stir in remaining ingredients. Pour into 9-inch square baking pan; freeze 3 hours or until firm. With electric mixer or food processor, beat mixture until smooth. Return to pan; freeze 6 hours or until

firm. Serve sorbet in Poached Pears, drizzled with Poached Pears syrup, or serve in stemmed glassware. Garnish, if desired, with fresh mint.

Poached Pears: In large skillet, thoroughly blend wine, sugar and lemon juice. Add pear halves, cut side down, and simmer covered 15 minutes or until pears are tender. Remove pears and chill. Cook remaining liquid, uncovered, over medium-high heat 10 minutes or until liquid is reduced by half; chill.

Nutrients per serving with Poached Pears:			
Calories	73	Sodium	4 mg
Fat	0 g	Cholesterol	0 mg

Nutrients per serving for Zinfandel Sorbet only:			
Calories	197	Sodium	7 mg
Fat	0 g	Cholesterol	0 mg

Raisin Streusel Bars

Low Cholesterol

Makes 12 bars

  2 cups KELLOGG'S® Raisin Bran cereal
  ¾ cup whole wheat flour
  ¾ cup all-purpose flour
  ¾ cup firmly packed brown sugar
  ¼ teaspoon salt
  ½ teaspoon baking soda
  ¼ teaspoon cinnamon
  ⅓ cup margarine, softened
  2 tablespoons water
  ½ cup strawberry preserves

Orange Glaze
  ½ cup powdered sugar
  1 teaspoon water
  3 tablespoons orange marmalade

1. In medium-size bowl, combine KELLOGG'S® Raisin Bran cereal, flours, brown sugar, salt, soda and cinnamon. Using pastry blender, cut in margarine until mixture resembles coarse crumbs. Stir in water. Set aside 1 cup of the cereal mixture. Press remaining mixture in bottom of greased 9×9×2-inch baking pan.

2. Spread strawberry preserves evenly over cereal mixture in bottom of pan. Sprinkle with reserved cereal mixture.

3. Bake in 350°F oven about 25 minutes or until lightly browned; cool completely.

4. To make glaze: Combine powdered sugar, water and marmalade until thoroughly combined. Drizzle over cooled bars.

Variation: ½ cup orange marmalade may be substituted for the strawberry preserves in this bar.

Nutrients per serving:			
Calories	240	Sodium	202 mg
Fat	5 g	Cholesterol	0 mg

Lite Marbled Angel Cake

Low Cholesterol

Makes 18 servings

1 box (14.5 ounces) angel food cake mix
¼ cup HERSHEY'S Cocoa
　Chocolate Glaze (recipe follows)

Adjust oven rack to lowest position. Heat oven to 375°. Prepare cake batter according to package directions. Measure 4 cups batter into separate bowl; gradually fold cocoa into this batter until well blended, being careful not to deflate batter. Alternately pour vanilla and chocolate batters into ungreased 10-inch tube pan. Cut through batter with knife or spatula to marble batter. Bake 30 to 35 minutes or until top crust is firm and looks very dry. Do not underbake. Cool, hanging pan upside down on heat-proof funnel or bottle, at least 1½ hours. Carefully run knife along side of pan to loosen cake. Place on serving plate; drizzle with Chocolate Glaze.

Chocolate Glaze: In small saucepan bring ⅓ cup sugar and ¼ cup water to full boil, stirring until sugar dissolves; remove from heat. Immediately add 1 cup HERSHEY'S® Mini Chips Semi-Sweet Chocolate; stir with wire whisk until chips are melted and mixture is smooth. Cool to desired consistency; use immediately. About ⅔ cup glaze.

Nutrients per serving:			
Calories	176	Sodium	114 mg
Fat	3 g	Cholesterol	0 mg

Luscious Lemon Bars

Low Sodium

Makes 2 dozen bars

Crust
　¼ cup CRISCO® Shortening
　¼ cup granulated sugar
　¼ teaspoon salt (optional)
　1 cup all-purpose flour
1½ teaspoons skim milk

Filling
　1 egg
　1 egg white
　1 cup granulated sugar
　2 teaspoons finely shredded fresh lemon peel
　3 tablespoons fresh lemon juice
　2 tablespoons all-purpose flour
　½ teaspoon baking powder

Drizzle
　¾ cup powdered sugar
　1 tablespoon skim milk
　½ teaspoon vanilla
　¼ teaspoon finely shredded fresh lemon peel

1. Heat oven to 350°F. Grease 8-inch square pan.

2. For crust: Place CRISCO® in large bowl. Beat at medium speed of electric mixer 30 seconds. Add granulated sugar and salt (if used). Beat until fluffy. Stir in flour and milk until crumbly and well mixed. Turn into pan. Press evenly against bottom.

3. Bake at 350°F for 15 minutes.

4. For filling: Combine egg, egg white, granulated sugar, lemon peel, lemon juice, flour and baking powder. Beat at high speed 3 minutes. Pour over hot, baked crust.

5. Bake at 350°F for 25 minutes or until light golden brown. Cool.

6. For drizzle: Combine powdered sugar, milk, vanilla and lemon peel. Drizzle over top. Allow to set before cutting into bars.

Nutrients per serving:			
Calories	100	Sodium	15 mg
Fat	2 g	Cholesterol	10 mg

Chocolate Pudding Parfaits

Low Sodium

Makes 6 servings

⅔ cup sugar
¼ cup HERSHEY'S® Cocoa
3 tablespoons cornstarch
　Dash salt
2 cups skim milk
1 tablespoon margarine
1 teaspoon vanilla
1 envelope (1.4 ounces) whipped topping mix
½ cup *cold* skim milk
¼ teaspoon vanilla
¼ teaspoon grated orange peel
　Orange slices (optional)

Combine sugar, cocoa, cornstarch and salt in medium saucepan; gradually stir in 2 cups milk. Cook over medium heat, stirring constantly, until mixture boils; boil and stir 1 minute. Remove from heat; blend in margarine and vanilla. Pour into medium bowl. Press plastic wrap onto surface of pudding; chill. Combine topping mix, cold milk and vanilla in small bowl; prepare according to package directions. Fold ½ cup whipped topping into pudding. Blend orange peel into remaining whipped topping. Alternately spoon chocolate pudding and orange flavored whipped topping into parfait glasses. Chill. Garnish with orange slices, if desired.

Nutrients per serving:			
Calories	176	Sodium	93 mg
Fat	4 g	Cholesterol	2 mg

Creamy Frozen Yogurt

Low Sodium

Makes 7 (½ cup) servings

1 package (4-serving size) JELL-O® Brand Sugar
    Free Gelatin, any flavor
1 cup boiling water
½ cup cold water
1 container (8 ounces) plain low fat yogurt
2 cups thawed COOL WHIP® Whipped Topping

Dissolve gelatin in boiling water. Add cold water. Stir in yogurt until well blended and smooth. Fold in whipped topping. Pour into 9-inch square pan. Freeze until firm, about 6 hours or overnight. Scoop into individual dessert dishes.

Nutrients per serving:			
Calories	80	Sodium	60 mg
Fat	4 g	Cholesterol	5 mg

Chocolate-Banana Cream Pie

Low Cholesterol

Makes 8 servings

¼ cup sugar
¼ cup cornstarch
2 tablespoons baking cocoa
2 cups cold skim milk
1 teaspoon vanilla
2 bananas, sliced
1 KEEBLER® Ready-Crust Chocolate Flavored
    pie crust
    Reduced-calorie whipped topping (optional)
    Additional banana slices for garnish (optional)

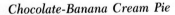

Chocolate-Banana Cream Pie

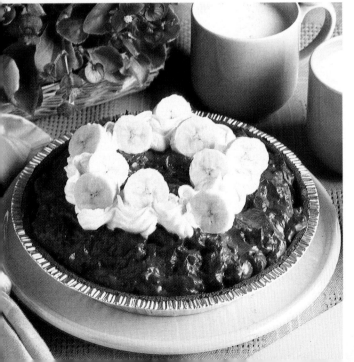

In a saucepan, combine sugar, cornstarch and cocoa. Whisk in cold milk. Cook over medium heat, stirring constantly until the mixture comes to a boil. Boil and stir 3 minutes. Remove from heat, stir in vanilla. Remove to a bowl, cover surface with plastic wrap. Refrigerate until cool, about 1 hour. Slice bananas into crust. Spoon cooled chocolate mixture over bananas. Cover with plastic wrap; press onto surface. Refrigerate at least 2 hours. Garnish with whipped topping and banana slices, if desired.

Nutrients per serving:			
Calories	213	Sodium	132 mg
Fat	6 g	Cholesterol	1 mg

Diet Chocolate Cheesecakes

Low Cholesterol

Makes 6 servings

1 packet unflavored gelatin
2 tablespoons skim milk
⅓ cup skim milk
2 tablespoons sugar
1½ tablespoons HERSHEY'S® Cocoa
¾ teaspoon vanilla
¾ cup low fat cottage cheese
1 egg white
1 tablespoon sugar
3 tablespoons graham cracker crumbs
    Dash cinnamon
    Fresh peach slices or naturally sweetened
    canned peach slices, drained (optional)

Sprinkle gelatin over 2 tablespoons skim milk in blender container; let stand several minutes to soften. Meanwhile, heat ⅓ cup skim milk to boiling; pour into blender container and process until gelatin dissolves. Add 2 tablespoons sugar, cocoa and the vanilla; process at medium speed until well blended. Add cottage cheese; blend at high speed until smooth. Pour into bowl; chill until mixture mounds from a spoon. Beat egg white until frothy; gradually add 1 tablespoon sugar and beat until stiff peaks form. Fold into chocolate mixture. Combine graham cracker crumbs and cinnamon; divide evenly among 6 paper-lined muffin cups (2½ inches in diameter). Divide chocolate mixture evenly among prepared cups. Cover; chill several hours or overnight. Serve garnished with peach slices, if desired.

Nutrients per serving:			
Calories	85	Sodium	153 mg
Fat	1 g	Cholesterol	3 mg

Toasted Almond Frozen Yogurt

Makes 6 servings

½ cup whole natural almonds
1½ cups lowfat milk
3 egg yolks
¾ cup sugar
1 cup lowfat plain yogurt
1 teaspoon vanilla
½ teaspoon almond extract
    Fresh fruit (optional)

Spread almonds in single layer on baking sheet. Bake at 350°F, 12 to 15 minutes, stirring occasionally, until lightly toasted. Cool; chop coarsely. Bring milk to a boil in heavy saucepan; set aside. Beat egg yolks with sugar until light and lemon colored. Gradually stir in hot milk; mix well. Return egg yolk mixture to pan. Cook, stirring constantly, over low heat until mixture coats back of spoon. Do not boil. Remove from heat and cool. Blend in yogurt, vanilla and almond extract. Stir in almonds. Pour mixture into ice cream freezer. Freeze according to manufacturer's directions. Serve with fresh fruit, if desired.

Nutrients per serving:			
Calories	252	Sodium	63 mg
Fat	10 g	Cholesterol	112 mg

Favorite recipe from **Almond Board of California**

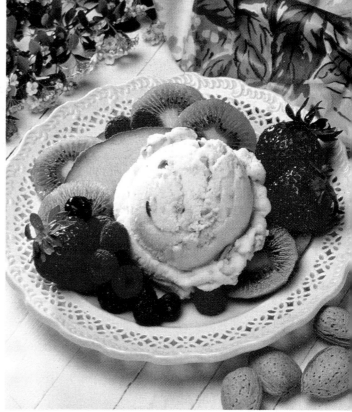

Toasted Almond Frozen Yogurt

Lemon Cheesecake Cups

Makes 6 servings

1 package (4-serving size) JELL-O® Brand Sugar
    Free Gelatin, Lemon Flavor
¾ cup boiling water
3 ounces light neufchatel cheese, softened and
    cut into cubes
½ cup cold water
1 teaspoon grated lemon rind (optional)
½ cup thawed COOL WHIP® Whipped Topping
    Graham cracker crumbs (optional)
    Lemon slices (optional)
    Mint leaves (optional)

Dissolve gelatin in boiling water in blender container; cover. Blend at medium speed 1 minute. Add cream cheese. Blend until smooth, about 1 minute. Add cold water and lemon rind. Cool slightly.

Blend whipped topping into gelatin mixture. Spoon into dessert dishes. Chill 1 hour. Sprinkle with graham cracker crumbs and garnish with lemon slices and mint leaves, if desired.

Nutrients per serving:			
Calories	60	Sodium	100 mg
Fat	5 g	Cholesterol	15 mg

Blueberry Blintzes

Makes 4 servings

¾ cup flour
⅓ teaspoon cinnamon
¾ cup LIGHT N' LIVELY® Skim Milk
2 tablespoons cold water

⅔ cup LIGHT N' LIVELY® Cottage Cheese
4 ozs. Light PHILADELPHIA BRAND®
    Neufchatel Cheese, softened
1 cup blueberries
1 tablespoon sugar

In small bowl of electric mixer, combine flour, cinnamon, milk and water, mixing at medium speed until smooth. Let stand 30 minutes. For each blintz, pour 3 tablespoons batter into hot, lightly greased 6-inch skillet or crepe pan. Cook on one side only until underside is lightly browned.

Preheat oven to 350°.

Combine remaining ingredients; mix lightly. Fill each blintz with ¼ cup cheese mixture; fold in sides and roll lengthwise. Place, seam side down, in 9-inch square pan. Bake 15 minutes. Garnish with additional blueberries and lime slices, if desired.

Nutrients per serving:			
Calories	230	Sodium	270 mg
Fat	8 g	Cholesterol	30 mg

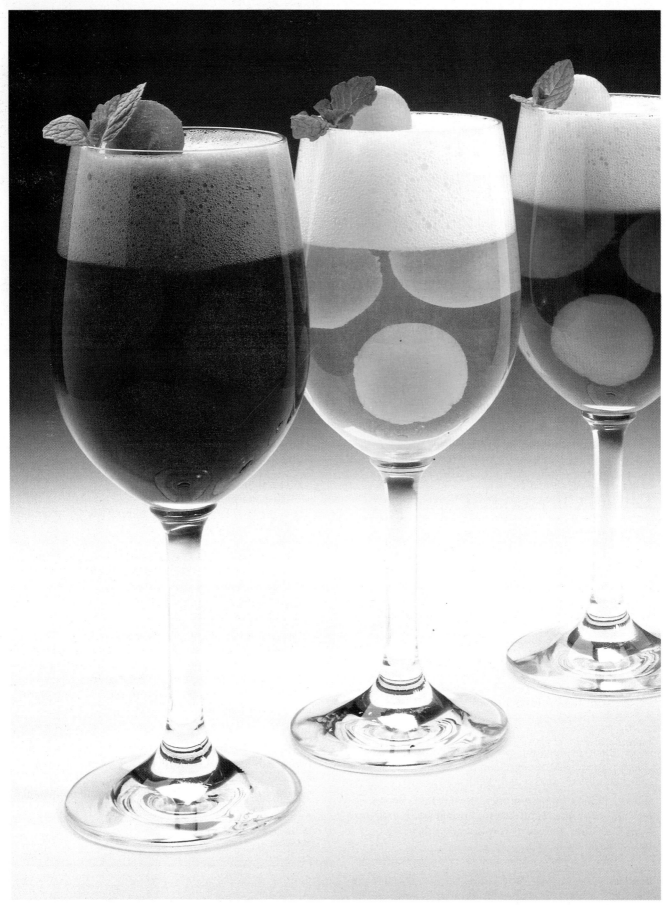

Melon Bubbles

Melon Bubbles

Makes 7 (½-cup) servings

1 package (4-serving size) JELL-O® Brand Sugar
    Free Gelatin, any flavor
¾ cup boiling water
½ cup cold water
    Ice cubes
1 cup melon balls (cantaloupe, honeydew or
    watermelon)
    Mint leaves (optional)

DISSOLVE gelatin in boiling water. Combine cold water and ice cubes to make 1¼ cups. Add to gelatin, stirring until slightly thickened. Remove any unmelted ice. Measure 1⅓ cups gelatin into small bowl; add melon. Pour into dessert dishes or serving bowl.

WHIP remaining gelatin at high speed of electric mixer until fluffy, thick and about doubled in volume. Spoon over gelatin in glasses. Chill until set, about 2 hours. Garnish with additional melon balls and mint leaves, if desired.

Nutrients per serving:

Calories	12	Sodium	35 mg
Fat	0 g	Cholesterol	0 mg

It's the Berries Pie

Makes 8 servings

1 quart fresh strawberries, washed and hulled,
    reserving 8 for garnish
1 KEEBLER® Ready-Crust Butter Flavored pie
    crust
1½ cups fresh or frozen raspberries (without sugar)
2 tablespoons sugar
1 package (0.3 ounces) triple berry or raspberry
    flavored sugar-free gelatin
1 cup boiling water
    Reduced-calorie whipped topping (optional)

Place prepared whole strawberries, hull side down, in the pie crust. Purée raspberries and sugar in blender or food processor. Press through a sieve to remove seeds. Set raspberry purée aside. Prepare gelatin according to package directions using 1 cup water. Chill until slightly thickened. Stir raspberry puree into gelatin and pour over strawberries. Chill until firm. Garnish with a dollop of whipped topping and a fresh berry, if desired.

Nutrients per serving:

Calories	164	Sodium	154 mg
Fat	5 g	Cholesterol	0 mg

Chocolate Chip Cookies

Makes 3 dozen cookies

2 cups all-purpose flour
1 teaspoon baking soda
½ teaspoon salt
1 egg
3 tablespoons water
1 teaspoon vanilla
1 cup firmly packed brown sugar
¼ cup PURITAN® Oil
½ cup semi-sweet chocolate chips

1. Heat oven to 375°F. Grease baking sheets well.

2. Combine flour, soda and salt. Set aside.

3. Combine egg, water and vanilla. Set aside.

4. Blend brown sugar and PURITAN® Oil in large bowl at low speed of electric mixer. Add egg mixture. Beat until smooth. Add flour mixture in three parts at lowest speed. Scrape bowl well after each addition. Stir in chocolate chips.

5. Drop dough by rounded teaspoonfuls onto baking sheets. Bake at 375°F for 7 to 8 minutes or until lightly browned. Cool on baking sheets 1 minute. Remove to cooling rack.

Nutrients per cookie:

Calories	80	Sodium	60 mg
Fat	2 g	Cholesterol	10 mg

Quick Chocolate Cupcakes

Makes 1½ dozen cupcakes

1½ cups unsifted all-purpose flour
1 cup sugar
¼ cup HERSHEY'S® Cocoa
1 teaspoon baking soda
½ teaspoon salt
1 cup water
¼ cup plus 2 tablespoons vegetable oil
1 tablespoon vinegar
1 teaspoon vanilla

Combine flour, sugar, cocoa, baking soda and salt in medium bowl. Add water, oil, vinegar and vanilla. Beat with mixer, wire whisk or wooden spoon until batter is smooth and ingredients are well blended. Pour batter into paper-lined muffin cups (2½ inches in diameter), filling each ⅔ full. Bake at 375° for 16 to 18 minutes or until tester inserted in center comes out clean. Remove to wire rack; cool completely. Frost as desired.

Nutrients per serving:

Calories	129	Sodium	121 mg
Fat	5 g	Cholesterol	0 mg

Health Nut Almond Oaties

Low Sodium

Makes 3 dozen cookies

¾ cup whole natural almonds
6 tablespoons margarine
1 cup brown sugar
½ cup granulated sugar
1 egg
1 teaspoon vanilla extract
¾ cup flour
1 teaspoon *each* baking soda and cinnamon
3½ cups old-fashioned rolled oats
1 can (8 ounces) crushed pineapple in juice
1 cup raisins

Spread almonds in single layer on baking sheet. Bake at 350°F, 12 to 15 minutes, stirring occasionally, until lightly toasted. Cool. Chop almonds and set aside. Beat margarine with brown sugar and granulated sugar until light and fluffy. Beat in egg and vanilla. Mix together flour, baking soda and cinnamon; stir into creamed mixture. Mix in oats, pineapple, raisins and reserved almonds. Drop dough by heaping tablespoonfuls onto lightly greased baking sheet. Flatten mounds with the back of a fork. Bake at 350°F, 10 to 12 minutes, until cookies are lightly browned. Remove to a wire rack to cool.

Nutrients per cookie:			
Calories	126	Sodium	51 mg
Fat	4 g	Cholesterol	8 mg

Favorite recipe from **Almond Board of California**

Health Nut Almond Oaties

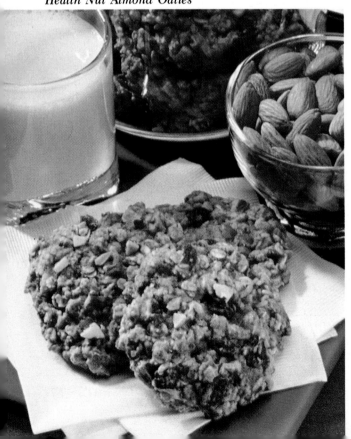

Individual Strawberry Shortcakes

Low Cholesterol

Makes 10 servings

Strawberry Mixture
4 cups fresh strawberries, washed, hulled and sliced
2 tablespoons granulated sugar

Shortcake Biscuits
1¾ cups all-purpose flour
1 tablespoon granulated sugar
1 tablespoon baking powder
½ teaspoon salt (optional)
¼ cup CRISCO® Shortening
⅔ cup milk

Topping
1 cup plain nonfat yogurt
3 tablespoons brown sugar
½ teaspoon vanilla

1. For strawberry mixture: Combine berries and sugar. Cover and refrigerate until ready to use.

2. Heat oven to 450°F.

3. For biscuits: Combine flour, sugar, baking powder and salt (if used) in bowl. Cut in CRISCO® with pastry blender (or 2 knives) until all flour is just blended to form coarse crumbs.

4. Add milk. Stir until dry ingredients are just moistened. Place on floured surface. Knead gently with fingertips 8 to 10 times. Pat or roll into 9-inch circle about ½-inch thick. (Hint: Cover dough with waxed paper. Press and flatten with 9-inch round cake pan until dough is desired thickness.)

5. Cut with 2½-inch round biscuit cutter. (Cut 7 biscuits; press dough scraps into ball and flatten again. Cut 3 biscuits.) Place on ungreased baking sheet.

6. Bake at 450°F for 12 minutes or until tops are golden brown.

7. For topping: Combine yogurt, brown sugar and vanilla. Stir gently until smooth.

8. To assemble: Split warm or cooled biscuits in half crosswise. Spoon about ¼ cup fruit over bottom half. Add tops. Spoon yogurt sauce over tops. Add another spoonful of fruit.

Nutrients per serving:			
Calories	197	Sodium	129 mg
Fat	6 g	Cholesterol	3 mg

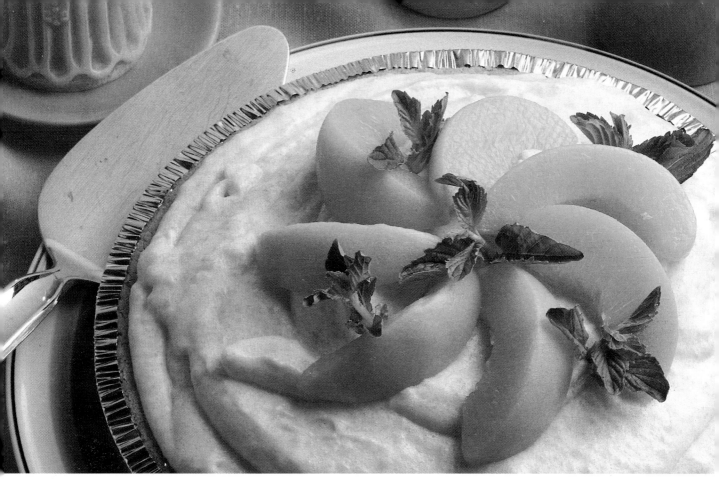

Light Peaches 'n Cream Pie

Light Peaches 'n Cream Pie

Low Cholesterol

Makes 8 servings

¼ cup cold water
2 packages unflavored gelatin
½ cup hot water
¼ cup sugar
2 cans (16 ounces *each*) sliced light peaches, drained
1 teaspoon vanilla
1 envelope whipped topping mix, prepared according to directions using skim milk
1 KEEBLER® Ready-Crust Graham Cracker pie crust
Reduced-calorie whipped topping (optional)
Peach slices for garnish

In blender container, add cold water. Sprinkle gelatin over water and blend on low. Let stand 3 to 4 minutes. Add hot water, cover and process until gelatin dissolves, about 2 minutes. Add sugar, peaches and vanilla. Cover and process until smooth. Pour into a mixing bowl. Chill until mixture begins to thicken. Fold whipped topping into peach mixture. Pour into crust. Chill 2 hours. Garnish with peach slices.

Nutrients per serving

Calories	233	Sodium	170 mg
Fat	8 g	Cholesterol	0 mg

Chocolate Cloud

Low Sodium

Makes 8 servings

1 envelope KNOX® Unflavored Gelatine
½ cup sugar
¼ cup unsweetened cocoa powder
2 eggs, separated
2 cups skim milk, divided
1½ teaspoons vanilla

In a medium saucepan, mix unflavored gelatine, sugar and cocoa powder; blend in egg yolks beaten with 1 cup milk. Let stand 1 minute. Stir over low heat until gelatine is completely dissolved, about 5 minutes. Stir in remaining 1 cup milk and vanilla. Pour into large bowl and chill, stirring occasionally, until mixture mounds slightly when dropped from spoon, about 1 hour.

In large bowl, beat egg whites until soft peaks form; gradually add gelatine mixture and beat until mixture doubles in volume, about 5 minutes. Chill until mixture is slightly thickened, about 30 minutes. Turn into 8 dessert dishes or 4-cup bowl; chill until set, about 1 hour.

Nutrients per serving:

Calories	102	Sodium	47 mg
Fat	2 g	Cholesterol	55 mg

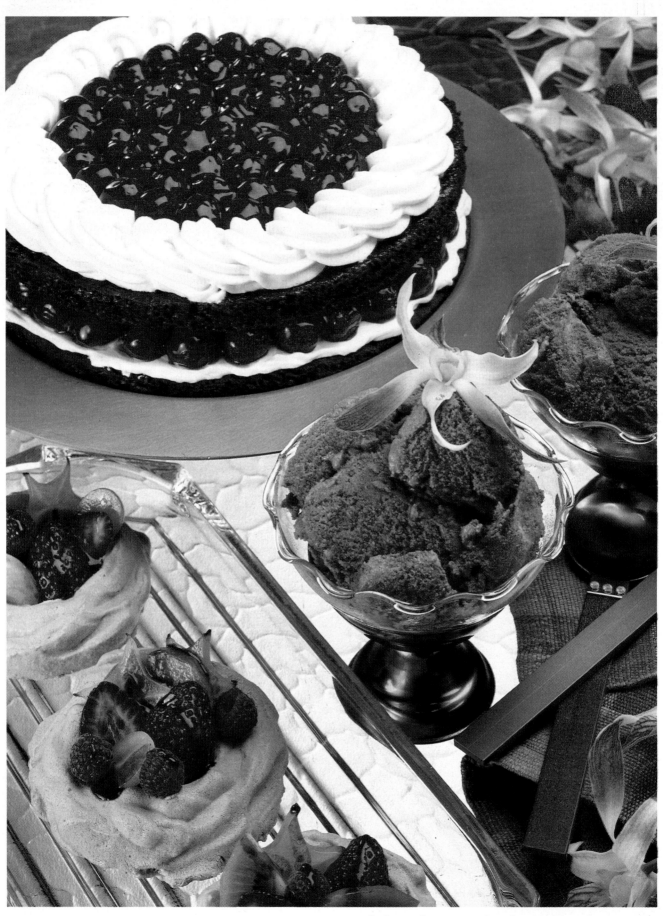

Clockwise from top: Chocolate Cherry Delight Cake,
Fruit Filled Chocolate Dreams and Caribbean Freeze

Chocolate Cherry Delight Cake

Low Cholesterol

Makes 12 servings

1 cup sugar
1 cup all-purpose flour
⅓ cup HERSHEY'S® Cocoa
¾ teaspoon baking soda
¾ teaspoon baking powder
   Dash salt
½ cup skim milk
¼ cup frozen egg substitute, thawed
¼ cup vegetable oil
1 teaspoon vanilla extract
½ cup boiling water
   Whipped Topping (recipe follows)
1 can (20 ounces) lower calorie cherry pie filling, chilled

Heat oven to 350°. Line bottom of 2 round 9 inch cake pans with wax paper. In large bowl combine sugar, flour, cocoa, baking soda, baking powder and salt. Add milk, egg substitute, oil and vanilla; beat on medium speed 2 minutes. Remove from mixer; stir in boiling water (batter will be thin). Pour into prepared pans. Bake 18 to 22 minutes or until wooden pick inserted in center comes out clean. Cool 10 minutes; remove from pans. Carefully remove wax paper. Cool completely. To assemble dessert, place one cake layer on serving plate. Spread with half Whipped Topping; top with half pie filling. Top with second layer. Spread with remaining topping and pie filling. Chill at least 1 hour.

Whipped Topping: In small, deep narrow-bottom bowl blend ½ cup cold skim milk, ½ teaspoon vanilla extract and 1 envelope (1.4 oz.) whipped topping mix. Whip at high speed with electric mixer until topping peaks, about 2 minutes. Continue beating 2 minutes longer until topping is light and fluffy.

Nutrients per serving:

Calories	220	Sodium	121 mg
Fat	6 g	Cholesterol	0 mg

Fruit Filled Chocolate Dreams

Low Cholesterol

Makes 5 servings

½ cup cold skim milk
½ teaspoon vanilla
1 envelope (1.4 oz.) whipped topping mix
1 tablespoon HERSHEY'S® Cocoa
   Assorted fresh fruit
   Chocolate Sauce (recipe follows)

In small deep narrow-bottom bowl blend cold skim milk, vanilla, topping mix and cocoa. Whip at high speed with electric mixer until topping peaks, about 2 minutes. Continue beating 2 minutes longer or until topping is light and fluffy. Spoon mixture into five mounds onto aluminum-foil-covered cookie sheet; with spoon, shape into shells. Freeze. To serve: Fill center of each frozen shell with fresh, cut-up fruit; drizzle with Chocolate Sauce.

Chocolate Sauce

¾ cup sugar
⅓ cup HERSHEY'S® Cocoa
1 tablespoon cornstarch
¾ cup water
1 tablespoon margarine
1 teaspoon vanilla

In small saucepan combine sugar, cocoa and cornstarch; stir in water. Cook over medium heat, stirring constantly, until mixture comes to a boil; boil 1 minute. Remove from heat; add margarine and vanilla, stirring until smooth. Chill thoroughly. Makes 1 cup.

Nutrients per serving (2 tablespoons sauce; does not include fresh fruit):

Calories	154	Sodium	31 mg
Fat	2 g	Cholesterol	0 mg

Caribbean Freeze

Low Sodium

Makes 4 servings

⅔ cup sugar
3 tablespoons HERSHEY'S® Cocoa
1¾ cups water
3 tablespoons frozen pineapple juice concentrate, thawed
2 teaspoons golden rum

In medium saucepan combine sugar and cocoa; stir in water. Cook over medium heat, stirring occasionally, until mixture comes to a boil; simmer 3 minutes. Cool to room temperature; stir in concentrate and rum. Chill. Pour chilled mixture into 1-quart container of ice cream freezer; freeze according to manufacturer's directions.

Nutrients per serving:

Calories	165	Sodium	2 mg
Fat	0 g	Cholesterol	0 mg

Acknowledgements

The publishers would like to thank the companies
and organizations listed below for the use of their
recipes in this book.

Almond Board of California
American Lamb Council
Armour Food Company
Blue Diamond Growers
Borden, Inc.
California Cling Peach Advisory Board
Campbell Soup Company
Carnation Company
Chef Paul Prudhomme's Magic Seasoning Blends™
Dole Packaged Foods Company
Heinz U.S.A.
Hershey Foods Corporation
Keebler Company
Kellogg Company
Kraft General Foods, Inc.

McIlhenny Company
National Fisheries Institute
National Live Stock and Meat Board
National Pork Producers Council
National Turkey Federation
Pet Incorporated
Pollio Dairy Products Corporation
The Procter & Gamble Company, Inc.
The Quaker Oats Company
StarKist Seafood Company
Swift-Eckrich, Inc.
Thomas J. Lipton, Inc.
United Fresh Fruit and Vegetable Association
Wisconsin Milk Marketing Board

Photo Credits

The publishers would like to thank the companies
and organizations listed below for the use of their
photographs in this book.

American Lamb Council
Armour Food Company
Borden, Inc.
Campbell Soup Company
Carnation Company
Dole Packaged Foods Company
Heinz U.S.A.
Hershey Foods Corporation
Keebler Company
Kellogg Company
Kraft General Foods, Inc.

McIlhenny Company
National Fisheries Institute
National Live Stock and Meat Board
National Pork Producers Council
Pollio Dairy Products Corporation
The Procter & Gamble Company, Inc.
The Quaker Oats Company
StarKist Seafood Company
Swift-Eckrich, Inc.
Thomas J. Lipton, Inc.

Index

Almonds
Almond Ratatouille, 65
Health Nut Almond Oaties, 88
Oriental Almond Stir-Fry, 35
Pan Roasted Herbed Almonds, 8
Red, Green & Gold Squash Platter, 59
Spicy Chicken Bites, 11
Toasted Almond Frozen Yogurt, 85

Appetizers (see also Dips & Spreads)
Chili-Cheese Wontons with Cilantro Sauce, 18
Confetti Tuna in Celery Sticks, 16
Ginger Shrimp, 7
Grilled Mushrooms with Lamb and Herbs, 17
Hot Dog Biscuit Bites, 8
Italian Bread Pizza, 15
Pan Roasted Herbed Almonds, 8
Party Ham Sandwiches, 8
Pineapple Shrimp Appetizers, 17
Scandinavian Smörgåsbord, 11
Shanghai Party Pleasers, 7
Spicy Chicken Bites, 11
Steamed Mussels in White Wine, 13
Tuna-Stuffed Artichokes, 14
Two-Tone Lite Ricotta Loaf, 10

Apples
Lemony Apple-Bran Salad, 70
Pork Curry, 56
Apple Streusel Coffee Cake, 32
Apricot Muffins, 29

Asparagus
Asparagus and Surimi Seafood Soup, 28
Scandinavian Smörgåsbord, 11

Bacon Pilaf, 66
Baked Tomatoes Florentine, 69
Baking Powder Biscuits, 32

Bananas
Banana Bran Loaf, 31
Bombay Banana Salad, 62
Caribbean Yam Bake, 68
Chicken Columbia, 56
Chocolate-Banana Cream Pie, 84
Curried Fruit and Rice Salad, 69
Frosty Juice Shake, 13
Orange-Banana Yogurt Dressing, 72
Refreshing Cocoa-Fruit Sherbet, 80
Strawberry-Banana Yogurt Dressing, 72

Summer Fruit Salad, 72
Barbecued Pork Chops, 54

Beef
Beef Cubed Steaks Provençale, 48
Butterflied Eye Round Roast, 57
Fast Beef Roast with Mushroom Sauce, 42
Herb-Marinated Chuck Steak, 49
Lasagna, 36
Minestrone, 30
Pizza Stuffed Peppers, 55
Southwestern Beef Stew, 35
Spaghetti Pizza Deluxe, 47
Stir-Fry Beef & Noodles, 52

Beverages
Choco-Berry Splash, 10
Chocolate Egg Cream, 14
Christmas Punch, 15
Cooler-Than-Cool Yogurt Drink, 15
Frosty Chocolate Shake, 19
Frosty Juice Shake, 13
Fruit Juice Combo, 12
Hot Curried V8, 9
Imperial Pineapple Nog, 19
Low-Calorie Lemonade, 14
Mexicali Sipper, 9
Pineapple Raspberry Punch, 9
Skim Milk Hot Cocoa, 12
Sparkling V8, 9
Strawberry Fizz, 11

Blueberries
Blueberry Blintzes, 85
Blueberry Lover's Muffins, 27
Blue Cheese Ball, 12
Bombay Banana Salad, 62

Breads
Apple Streusel Coffee Cake, 32
Banana Bran Loaf, 31
Bran Pita Bread, 30
Common Sense™ Oat Bran Bread, 29
Orange Chocolate Chip Bread, 29
Pumpkin Patch Bread, 29
Touch of Honey Bread, 25
V8 Cheese Bread, 21

Broccoli
Broccoli Tarragon Soup, 24
Creamettes® Chicken Salad, 60
Light Pasta Salad, 60
Rotini Stir-Fry, 46
Stir-Fry Beef & Noodles, 52
Brunch Potato Cassoulet, 37
Butterflied Eye Round Roast, 57

Cakes (see also Cheesecakes)
Carrot Raisin Cake, 76
Cherry Angel Rolls, 75
Chocolate Cherry Delight Cake, 91
French Vanilla Fruit Delight, 80
Fudge Cake with Melba Topping, 76

Individual Strawberry Shortcakes, 88
Lite Marbled Angel Cake, 83
Peachy Snack Cake, 80
Quick Chocolate Cupcakes, 87
California Fruit Salad Rosé, 71
Caribbean Freeze, 91
Caribbean Yam Bake, 68

Carrots
Carrot Lemon Soup, 24
Carrot Raisin Cake, 76
Chilled Carrot Soup, 23
Harvest Bowl Soup, 21
Rotini Stir-Fry, 46
Springtime Vegetable Slaw, 70
Cashew-Shrimp Salad, 66

Casseroles
Brunch Potato Cassoulet, 37
Lasagna, 36
Spaghetti Pizza Deluxe, 47

Cheese
Baked Tomatoes Florentine, 69
Blueberry Blintzes, 85
Blue Cheese Ball, 12
Chili-Cheese Wontons with Cilantro Sauce, 18
Citrus Cheese Salad, 72
Dieter's Fish and Spinach, 38
Italian Bread Pizza, 15
Jalapeño Chicken Fajitas, 45
Lasagna, 36
Pizza Stuffed Peppers, 55
Rosy Blue Cheese Dressing, 64
Spaghetti Pizza Deluxe, 47
Stuffed Chicken Breasts, 41
Tacos de Queso, 37
Two-Cheese Enchiladas, 40
Two-Tone Lite Ricotta Loaf, 10
V8 Cheese Bread, 21

Cheesecakes
Creamy Lemon Cheesecake, 79
Diet Chocolate Cheesecakes, 84
Lemon Cheesecake Cups, 85
Cherry Angel Rolls, 75

Chicken
Baked Tomatoes Florentine, 69
Chicken Cilantro Bisque, 23
Chicken Columbia, 56
Chicken Lemon Soup Oriental, 33
Chicken Mushroom Crepes, 51
Chicken Pasta, 44
Creamettes® Chicken Salad, 60
Herb-Marinated Chicken Breasts, 38
Herb-Marinated Chicken Kabobs, 46
Jalapeño Chicken Fajitas, 45
Pepper-Chicken Fettuccini Toss, 41
Rotini Stir-Fry, 46
Spicy Chicken Bites, 11
Stuffed Chicken Breasts, 41
Sweet Sour Chicken Sauté, 40

Chili-Cheese Wontons with Cilantro
  Sauce, 18
Chilled Carrot Soup, 23
Choco-Berry Splash, 10
Chocolate
  Caribbean Freeze, 91
  Choco-Berry Splash, 10
  Chocolate-Banana Cream Pie, 84
  Chocolate Cherry Delight Cake, 91
  Chocolate Chip Cookies, 87
  Chocolate Cloud, 89
  Chocolate Egg Cream, 14
  Chocolate Pudding Parfaits, 83
  Chocolate Sauce, 91
  Diet Chocolate Cheesecakes, 84
  Frosty Chocolate Shake, 19
  Fruit Filled Chocolate Dreams, 91
  Lite Chocolate Sauce, 79
  Lite Marbled Angel Cake, 83
  Orange Chocolate Chip Bread, 29
  Quick Chocolate Cupcakes, 87
  Refreshing Cocoa-Fruit Sherbet,
    80
  Skim Milk Hot Cocoa, 12
Christmas Punch, 15
Cinnamon Fruit Tart with Sour
  Cream Filling, 77
Citrus Cheese Salad, 72
Colorful Cauliflower Bake, 68
Common Sense™ Oat Bran Bread, 29
Confetti Rice Salad, 62
Confetti Scallops & Noodles, 36
Confetti Tuna in Celery Sticks, 16
Cookies
  Chocolate Chip Cookies, 87
  Health Nut Almond Oaties, 88
  Luscious Lemon Bars, 83
  Oatmeal Raisin Cookies, 80
  Raisin Streusel Bars, 82
  Spice Cookies, 78
Cool Desserts
  Chocolate Cloud, 89
  Chocolate Pudding Parfaits, 83
  Jell-O® Sugar Free Jigglers Gelatin
    Snacks, 78
  Melon Bubbles, 87
  Strawberries 'n Cream Fool, 79
Cooler-Than-Cool Yogurt Drink, 15
Corn
  Corn Olé, 66
  Seafood Corn Chowder, 28
  Southwest Vegetable Chili, 39
Cranberry Oat Bran Muffins, 22
Creamettes® Chicken Salad, 60
Creamy Chili Dip, 16
Creamy Frozen Yogurt, 84
Creamy Fruit Mold, 71
Creamy Lemon Cheesecake, 79
Creamy V8 Dressing, 64
Crispened New Potatoes, 70

Cuban Black Bean & Ham Soup, 31
Cucumbers
  Cashew-Shrimp Salad, 66
  Cucumbers and Onions, 59
  Orange Roughy with Cucumber
    Relish, 39
  Pineapple Shrimp Appetizers, 17
Curried Fruit and Rice Salad, 69

Desserts: *see under* **Cakes,**
    Cheesecakes, Cookies, Cool
    Desserts, Frozen Desserts
    and **Pies & Tarts**
Diet Chocolate Cheesecakes, 84
Dieter's Fish and Spinach, 38
Dips & Spreads
  Blue Cheese Ball, 12
  Creamy Chili Dip, 16
  Eggplant Caviar, 19
  Garden Vegetable Dip, 18
  Lemony Fruit Dip, 18
  Ratatouille Appetizer, 16
Double Oat Muffins, 27

Easy Tuna Melt, 52
Eggplant
  Almond Ratatouille, 65
  Eggplant Caviar, 19
  Eggplant Italiano, 73
  Greek Lamb Sauté with
    Mostaccioli, 55
  Ratatouille Appetizer, 16

Family Baked Bean Dinner, 73
Fast Beef Roast with Mushroom
  Sauce, 42
Fish & Seafood
  Asparagus and Surimi Seafood
    Soup, 28
  Cashew-Shrimp Salad, 66
  Confetti Scallops & Noodles, 36
  Confetti Tuna in Celery Sticks, 16
  Dieter's Fish and Spinach, 38
  Easy Tuna Melt, 52
  Ginger Shrimp, 7
  "Grilled" Tuna with Vegetables in
    Herb Butter, 47
  Light 'n' Saucy Shrimp, 57
  Linguine with White Clam Sauce,
    48
  Orange Roughy with Cucumber
    Relish, 39
  Oriental Almond Stir-Fry, 35
  Oven Campout Fish with BBQ
    Sauce, 37
  Oven Crisped Fish, 49
  Pineapple Shrimp Appetizers, 17
  Scandinavian Smörgåsbord, 11
  Seafood Corn Chowder, 28
  Seafood Gumbo, 22

  Shrimp Creole, 54
  Spiced Broiled Lobster, 52
  Steamed Mussels in White Wine,
    13
  Tuna & Fresh Fruit Salad, 68
  Tuna-Lettuce Bundles, 48
  Tuna-Stuffed Artichokes, 14
  Tuna Tacos, 50
  Tuna Veronique, 40
  West Coast Bouillabaisse, 26
French Vanilla Fruit Delight, 80
Frosty Chocolate Shake, 19
Frosty Juice Shake, 13
Frozen Desserts
  Caribbean Freeze, 91
  Creamy Frozen Yogurt, 84
  Fruit Filled Chocolate Dreams, 91
  Refreshing Cocoa-Fruit Sherbet,
    80
  Toasted Almond Frozen Yogurt, 85
  Very Berry Sorbet, 75
  Zinfandel Sorbet with Poached
    Pears, 82
Fruit Juice Combo, 12
Fudge Cake with Melba Topping, 76

Garden Potato Soup, 24
Garden Vegetable Dip, 18
Ginger Shrimp, 7
Ginger-Soy Dressing, 64
Greek Lamb Sauté with Mostaccioli,
  55
Grilled Mushrooms with Lamb and
  Herbs, 17
"Grilled" Tuna with Vegetables in
  Herb Butter, 47

Ham
  Brunch Potato Cassoulet, 37
  Cuban Black Bean & Ham Soup,
    31
  Ham Breakfast Sandwich, 57
  Ham Tortellini Salad, 65
  Italian Bread Pizza, 15
  Party Ham Sandwiches, 8
  Vegetable and Ham Soup, 32
  Zesty Pasta Salad, 59
Harvest Bowl Soup, 21
Health Nut Almond Oaties, 88
Herb-Marinated Chicken Breasts, 38
Herb-Marinated Chicken Kabobs, 46
Herb-Marinated Chuck Steak, 49
Holiday Stir-Fry, 63
Honey
  Imperial Pineapple Nog, 19
  Lite Honey Mustard Dressing, 63
  Papaya Muffins, 33
  Touch of Honey Bread, 25
Hot Curried V8, 9
Hot Dog Biscuit Bites, 8

Imperial Pineapple Nog, 19
Individual Strawberry Shortcakes, 88
Italian Bread Pizza, 15
It's the Berries Pie, 87

Jalapeño Chicken Fajitas, 45
Jell-O® Sugar Free Jigglers Gelatin Snacks, 78

Lamb
Greek Lamb Sauté with Mostaccioli, 55
Grilled Mushrooms with Lamb and Herbs, 17
Lasagna, 36
Legumes
Cuban Black Bean & Ham Soup, 31
Family Baked Bean Dinner, 73
Harvest Bowl Soup, 21
Minestrone, 30
Southwest Vegetable Chili, 39
Tacos de Queso, 37
Lemon Cheesecake Cups, 85
Lemony Apple-Bran Salad, 70
Lemony Fruit Dip, 18
Light and Easy Turkey Tenderloins, 55
Light 'n' Saucy Shrimp, 57
Light Pasta Salad, 60
Light Peaches 'n Cream Pie, 89
Linguine with White Clam Sauce, 48
Lite Chocolate Sauce, 79
Lite Honey Mustard Dressing, 63
Lite Marbled Angel Cake, 83
Low-Calorie Lemonade, 14
Luscious Lemon Bars, 83

Melon Bubbles, 87
Mexicali Sipper, 9
Microwave Recipes
Almond Ratatouille, 65
Bacon Pilaf, 66
Barbecued Pork Chops, 54
Creamy Lemon Cheesecake, 79
Double Oat Muffins, 27
Family Baked Bean Dinner, 73
Pasta Primavera, 45
Poached Turkey Tenderloins with Tarragon Sauce, 42
Red, Green & Gold Squash Platter, 59
Shrimp Creole, 54
Stuffed Italian Zucchini, 64
Vegetable and Ham Soup, 32
Minestrone, 30
Muffins & Rolls
Apricot Muffins, 29
Baking Powder Biscuits, 32

Blueberry Lover's Muffins, 27
Cranberry Oat Bran Muffins, 22
Double Oat Muffins, 27
Papaya Muffins, 33
Whole Wheat Biscuits, 25
Mushrooms
Baked Tomatoes Florentine, 69
Chicken Lemon Soup Oriental, 33
Chicken Mushroom Crepes, 51
Grilled Mushrooms with Lamb and Herbs, 17
Mushroom Sauce, 42
Oriental Almond Stir-Fry, 35
Pepper-Chicken Fettuccini Toss, 41
Spaghetti Pizza Deluxe, 47
Stir-Fry Beef & Noodles, 52
Tuna-Stuffed Artichokes, 14

Oatmeal Raisin Cookies, 80
Orange-Banana Yogurt Dressing, 72
Orange Chocolate Chip Bread, 29
Orange Roughy with Cucumber Relish, 39
Oriental Almond Stir-Fry, 35
Oven Campout Fish with BBQ Sauce, 37
Oven Crisped Fish, 49

Pan Roasted Herbed Almonds, 8
Papaya Muffins, 33
Party Ham Sandwiches, 8
Pasta
Chicken Pasta, 44
Confetti Scallops & Noodles, 36
Creamettes® Chicken Salad, 60
Greek Lamb Sauté with Mostaccioli, 55
Ham Tortellini Salad, 65
Lasagna, 36
Light Pasta Salad, 60
Linguine with White Clam Sauce, 48
Minestrone, 30
Pasta Primavera, 45
Pepper-Chicken Fettuccini Toss, 41
Rotini Stir-Fry, 46
Spaghetti Pizza Deluxe, 47
Spaghetti with Pesto Sauce, 38
Stir-Fry Beef & Noodles, 52
Zesty Pasta Salad, 59
Peaches
Chicken Lemon Soup Oriental, 33
Confetti Rice Salad, 62
Fudge Cake with Melba Topping, 76
Light Peaches 'n Cream Pie, 89
Peachy Snack Cake, 80
Pears
Zinfandel Sorbet with Poached Pears, 82

Pepper-Chicken Fettuccini Toss, 41
Pies & Tarts
Chocolate-Banana Cream Pie, 84
Cinnamon Fruit Tart with Sour Cream Filling, 77
It's the Berries Pie, 87
Light Peaches 'n Cream Pie, 89
Pineapple
Christmas Punch, 15
Family Baked Bean Dinner, 73
Italian Bread Pizza, 15
Oven Campout Fish with BBQ Sauce, 37
Pineapple Shrimp Appetizers, 17
Shanghai Party Pleasers, 7
Summer Fruit Salad, 72
Warm Turkey Salad, 63
Pizza Stuffed Peppers, 55
Poached Turkey Tenderloins with Tarragon Sauce, 42
Pork (see also **Ham**)
Barbecued Pork Chops, 54
Pork Curry, 56
Pork Loin Roulade, 44
Saucy Pork and Peppers, 53
Potatoes
Brunch Potato Cassoulet, 37
Crispened New Potatoes, 70
Garden Potato Soup, 24
Pumpkin
Pumpkin Patch Bread, 29
Turkey Wild Rice Pumpkin Soup, 26

Quick Chocolate Cupcakes, 87

Raisin Streusel Bars, 82
Raspberries
Fudge Cake with Melba Topping, 76
It's the Berries Pie, 87
Pineapple Raspberry Punch, 9
Spinach Salad with Raspberry Dressing, 73
Ratatouille Appetizer, 16
Red, Green & Gold Squash Platter, 59
Refreshing Cocoa-Fruit Sherbet, 80
Rice
Bacon Pilaf, 66
Confetti Rice Salad, 62
Curried Fruit and Rice Salad, 69
Light n' Saucy Shrimp, 57
Seafood Gumbo, 22
Shrimp Creole, 54
Turkey Wild Rice Pumpkin Soup, 26
Wild Rice Sauté, 60
Rosy Blue Cheese Dressing, 64
Rotini Stir-Fry, 46

Salad Dressings
Creamy V8 Dressing, 64
Ginger-Soy Dressing, 64
Lite Honey Mustard Dressing, 63
Orange-Banana Yogurt Dressing, 72
Rosy Blue Cheese Dressing, 64
Strawberry-Banana Yogurt Dressing, 72
Thousand Island Dressing, 62
Yogurt Dressing, 59

Salads
Bombay Banana Salad, 62
California Fruit Salad Rosé, 71
Cashew-Shrimp Salad, 66
Citrus Cheese Salad, 72
Confetti Rice Salad, 62
Creamettes® Chicken Salad, 60
Creamy Fruit Mold, 71
Curried Fruit and Rice Salad, 69
Ham Tortellini Salad, 65
Lemony Apple-Bran Salad, 70
Light Pasta Salad, 60
Spinach Salad with Raspberry Dressing, 73
Springtime Vegetable Slaw, 70
Summer Fruit Salad, 72
Tuna & Fresh Fruit Salad, 68
Vegetable-Bulgur Salad, 61
Warm Turkey Salad, 63
Zesty Pasta Salad, 59

Sandwiches
Easy Tuna Melt, 52
Ham Breakfast Sandwich, 57
Jalapeño Chicken Fajitas, 45
Party Ham Sandwiches, 8
Tacos de Queso, 37
Tuna Tacos, 50

Sauces
Chocolate Sauce, 91
Lite Chocolate Sauce, 79
Mushroom Sauce, 42
Tarragon Sauce, 42
Saucy Pork and Peppers, 53
Scandinavian Smörgåsbord, 11

Seafood: *see under* **Fish & Seafood**
Shanghai Party Pleasers, 7
Shrimp Creole, 54
Skim Milk Hot Cocoa, 12

Soups
Asparagus and Surimi Seafood Soup, 28
Broccoli Tarragon Soup, 24
Carrot Lemon Soup, 24
Chicken Cilantro Bisque, 23
Chicken Lemon Soup Oriental, 33
Chilled Carrot Soup, 23
Cuban Black Bean & Ham Soup, 31
Garden Potato Soup, 24
Harvest Bowl Soup, 21

Minestrone, 30
Seafood Corn Chowder, 28
Seafood Gumbo, 22
Turkey Wild Rice Pumpkin Soup, 26
Vegetable and Ham Soup, 32
West Coast Bouillabaisse, 26
Southwestern Beef Stew, 35
Southwest Vegetable Chili, 39
Spaghetti Pizza Deluxe, 47
Spaghetti with Pesto Sauce, 38
Sparkling V8, 9
Spice Cookies, 78
Spiced Broiled Lobster, 52
Spicy Chicken Bites, 11

Spinach
Confetti Scallops & Noodles, 36
Dieter's Fish and Spinach, 38
Holiday Stir-Fry, 63
Spinach Salad with Raspberry Dressing, 73
Springtime Vegetable Slaw, 70
Steamed Mussels in White Wine, 13
Stir-Fry Beef & Noodles, 52

Strawberries
Choco-Berry Splash, 10
Christmas Punch, 15
Individual Strawberry Shortcakes, 88
It's the Berries Pie, 87
Strawberries 'n Cream Fool, 79
Strawberry-Banana Yogurt Dressing, 72
Strawberry Fizz, 11
Summer Fruit Salad, 72
Very Berry Sorbet, 75
Stuffed Chicken Breasts, 41
Stuffed Italian Zucchini, 64
Summer Fruit Salad, 72
Sweet 'n Sour Stir-Fry, 71
Sweet Sour Chicken Sauté, 40

Tacos de Queso, 37
Tarragon Sauce, 42
Thousand Island Dressing, 62
Toasted Almond Frozen Yogurt, 85

Tomatoes
Bacon Pilaf, 66
Baked Tomatoes Florentine, 69
Beef Cubed Steaks Provençale, 48
Corn Olé, 66
Ham Tortellini Salad, 65
Light n' Saucy Shrimp, 57
Minestrone, 30
Party Ham Sandwiches, 8
Pasta Primavera, 45
Saucy Pork and Peppers, 53
Seafood Gumbo, 22
Tuna Tacos, 50
West Coast Bouillabaisse, 26

Touch of Honey Bread, 25
Tuna & Fresh Fruit Salad, 68
Tuna-Lettuce Bundles, 48
Tuna-Stuffed Artichokes, 14
Tuna Tacos, 50
Tuna Veronique, 40

Turkey
Light and Easy Turkey Tenderloins, 55
Poached Turkey Tenderloins with Tarragon Sauce, 42
Shanghai Party Pleasers, 7
Turkey Wild Rice Pumpkin Soup, 26
Turkey with Orange Sauce, 53
Warm Turkey Salad, 63
Two-Cheese Enchiladas, 40
Two-Tone Lite Ricotta Loaf, 10

Vegetable and Ham Soup, 32
V8 Cheese Bread, 21
Vegetable-Bulgur Salad, 61

Vegetable Dishes
Almond Ratatouille, 65
Baked Tomatoes Florentine, 69
Caribbean Yam Bake, 68
Colorful Cauliflower Bake, 68
Corn Olé, 66
Crispened New Potatoes, 70
Cucumbers and Onions, 59
Eggplant Italiano, 73
Family Baked Bean Dinner, 73
Holiday Stir-Fry, 63
Red, Green & Gold Squash Platter, 59
Stuffed Italian Zucchini, 64
Sweet 'n Sour Stir-Fry, 71
Very Berry Sorbet, 75

Warm Turkey Salad, 63
West Coast Bouillabaisse, 26
Whole Wheat Biscuits, 25
Wild Rice Sauté, 60

Yogurt Dressing, 59

Zesty Pasta Salad, 59
Zinfandel Sorbet with Poached Pears, 82

Zucchini
Almond Ratatouille, 65
Beef Cubed Steaks Provençale, 48
Corn Olé, 66
Harvest Bowl Soup, 21
Herb-Marinated Chicken Kabobs, 46
Minestrone, 30
Red, Green & Gold Squash Platter, 59
Stuffed Italian Zucchini, 64

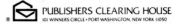